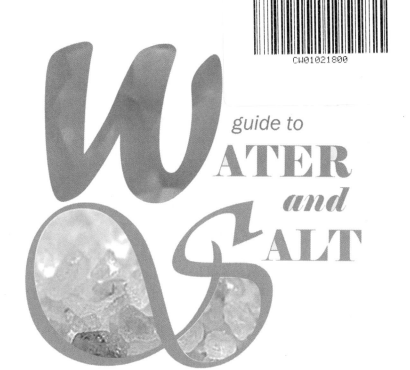

guide to

WATER
and
SALT

F. Batmanghelidj MD
Phillip Day

The Essential Guide to Water and Salt

Printing history

First edition	2008
Second edition	2014

ISBN 1-904015-22-0

Manufactured in Great Britain
Credence Publications
PO Box 3
TONBRIDGE
Kent TN12 9ZY UK
www.credence.org

WARNING: The information contained in this book is for
information purposes only and should not be construed as
medical advice for an individual's given condition. A medical
practitioner's qualified opinion should always be sought in the
matter of serious illness.

2nd ed.

Table of contents

Dedication and Thanks

This book is dedicated to the memory of Dr Fereydoon Batmanghelidj who passed away unexpectedly in November 2004. An obituary containing an assessment of his extraordinary life can be read on the Tagman Press website at www.tagman-press.com and on Dr B's original website, www.watercure.com, which will continue to be the main international focus for the mission being continued by his estate and family.

Special thanks go to Mrs Xiaopo Batmanghelidj for commissioning this book. Many thanks also go to the indefatigable Anthony Grey, founder of Tagman Press. Also to Sheryl McMillan, Steve Russell, Philip Smart in Japan and Samantha Day in the UK for the artwork and endless supplies of water during this work's compilation!

PD

Foreword

*'I know that most men, including those at ease with problems of the greatest complexity, can seldom accept even the simplest and most obvious truth if it would oblige them to admit the falsity of conclusions which they have delighted in explaining to colleagues, proudly taught to others, and which they have woven, thread by thread, into the fabric of their lives.' - **Leo Tolstoy***

Water and salt are essential to life. Intuitively, everyone knows it. We were born out of a water and salt sack. From our youngest years when we first accepted that cattle die without water and salt, the importance of these most elemental ingredients to our own existence has been entrenched in the human psyche. Books, TV and cinema remind that a man cannot cross a desert without water. An astronaut cannot venture into space without water. A human may survive longer than a month and a half without solid foods to sustain him, but without water he is finished within days. When we're cremated, all that is left is salt.

The fact that water and salt can heal the sick has been an ongoing wrangle in scientific circles for years, not because there's any doubt about it, but because no-one wants to spend fortunes funding studies if the only thing they have to sell at the end is salt and two atoms of hydrogen and one of oxygen. Ever since John Rockefeller and Abraham Flexner set up the modern medical system and doctors became 'licensed' to prescribe and sell patented chemicals, the nutrients of nature which daily sustain our bodies have been belittled in favour of the profitable pill as the panacea for all man's ills. Even today, how your doctor is trained and what he has been taught to tell and prescribe you bears more relation to economics than what will actually heal. Sickness is big business. No-one's making much money out of 'health' these days.

But deadlocks can be broken, though it sometimes takes an extraordinary man, placed in an extraordinary situation, to bring the world to its senses. The extraordinary man in this case is Iranian physician, Dr Fereydoon Batmanghelidj. The extraordinary situation was the two and a half years he spent in an Iranian prison following his arrest by the revolutionary mullahs after the Shah's overthrow. What Dr B discovered while tending the sick in Evin Prison, Tehran, is still causing ructions, and long may they continue until the world knows it. *Water heals! Perhaps you're not sick, you're just dehydrated! There is no system or function of the body not pegged to the flow of water!*

Think about it. We're told that salt is evil and yet don't question why severely sick people are put on a saline drip. The authorities deride any notion that the world is chronically dehydrated, yet there's a pub or bar on every corner. We're told that one beverage is as good as another (Coke machines in hospital corridors??), and that fluids are what count. The idea that water could be pharmacologically or even biophysically active and cure disease is, alas, nonsense to the university-trained MD. 'We'd have been told about it!' is the churlish response, angry that anyone could question the whole approach to symptom-based medicine.

Well, like you I'm a citizen and the end-user of all this 'medicine' and I'm not happy about it. Modern 'disease management' has cost many members of my family their lives and I'm *so* not happy about it, ten years ago I formed the Campaign for Truth in Medicine to inform the public of this medical quackery. I obviously touched a nerve since today the Campaign boasts a membership of thousands worldwide - many of them doctors - all pushing for a change in the way we view disease. Dr James Le Fanu's comment in the Sunday Telegraph sums up the current, hapless approach:

'The commonest misunderstanding in medicine is why doctors should 'treat the symptoms and not the cause', to which the response can only be that

5

regrettably, the cause of virtually every illness in the medical textbooks, from asthma and arthritis all the way to Zoons balanitis, is quite unknown. Thus the best we can hope for is to 'treat the symptoms' as effectively as we can.'[1]

Imagine that. *They don't know what causes disease....*

Dr Batmanghelidj's amazing work came across my desk during my own global crusade, and his writings struck a chord with my own. Certainly, doctors are not evil or wicked people; their commendable strides in progress should be given all credit where due. Infant survivability at birth. A & E trauma medicine. Diagnosis. Prosthesis. Within the realm of 'disease' and 'mental health', however, we see *utter failure*. In most industrialised nations, doctors are now the third leading cause of death – America the exception, where they are the leading cause of fatality.[2] The simple fact is, clearing symptoms with drugs is not the same thing as curing disease. Millions have been maimed or killed by chemotherapy and radiation for cancer over the years. Millions more are hooked on benzodiazepines and anti-depressants for invented conditions, drugged up in the belief they are suffering 'chemical imbalances' only drugs can solve.[3] What happened to our civilisation, our children, our grandparents, those we say we care the most about? Let me tell you what happened. We abrogated responsibility for protecting our own health and freedoms and surrendered them to others. And, as the saying goes, 'power corrupts, and absolute power corrupts absolutely'. Today we have the 'healthcare' system we deserve because most of us still don't want to take responsibility for how we live our lives.

Enter the extraordinary man. Perhaps posterity will one day accord Dr Batmanghelidj the honour he deserves for giving us back the

---

[1] *Sunday Telegraph*, 22nd October 2006,

[2] www.credence.org, search under 'gary null'

[3] Day, Phillip *The Mind Game*, Credence Publications, 2003

simple in medicine; Fleming and Koch never made such a contribution! Walk into any medical college, stare at the portraits in those hallowed halls of academia and be struck by one thing. Few, if any of those men and women were taught nutrition, hydration and the implications of lifestyle on health. Walk into any hospital at lunchtime today and it is clear they still don't teach them. *You are what you eat. What you drink. What you breathe in, slap on your skin, look at and listen to.* In fact, you are the sum total of everything you've ever done to yourself. Think about that next time you celebrate the fact that you are a water and salt being. Perhaps even raise a glass of the pure stuff in memory of that young doctor in Tehran, cast into prison long ago under sentence of death, wondering what on earth he could do to help anyone, let alone himself, with the little time he had left. A tale of how, in our technocratic age where science and money became gods and the simple truths escaped becoming known. Real water and real salt heal. How and why they do is the miracle contained in this book.

Phillip Day
Campaign for Truth in Medicine
www.credence.org

Introduction

Dr Batmanghelidj: After my training at St Mary's Hospital Medical School of London University, and having the honour of being selected as one of the resident doctors in my own medical school, I returned to Iran, where I was born, to set up medical centres and clinics for those in need. This endeavour became very successful - until the political volcano erupted as the angry masses engaged in the violent overthrow of the Shah and Iranian government.

And there was a tragic side to this historic event. Almost all the professional and creative people who had stayed in the country were rounded up and taken to prison to be investigated, tried and dealt with as quickly as possible. Some were shot on the first day or two. Their revolutionary trials consisted simply of establishment of identity and pronouncement of guilt, followed by sentence. The trial would last no more than ten minutes. Others were given a little more time before being processed.

I was lucky to be among the latter group. I suppose my skills as a doctor were useful to the prison authorities, explaining the delay in my being processed.

Evin Prison in Tehran, where I was held for two years and seven months, was built for 600 persons. At one point, it was 'sardine-packed' with 8,000 to 9,000 people. At the height of revolutionary fervour, when segregating different political factions, the authorities used cells built for six to eight to isolate up to 90 people. One third would lie down, one third would squat and one third had to stand. Every few hours, the prisoners would rotate position.

The nightmare of life and death in that hell-hole haunted everyone and tested the mettle of both strong and weak. This was when the human body revealed to me some of its greatest secrets - secrets never understood by the medical profession.

For most of the prisoners, who ranged in age from 14 to 80, the pressures of the exceptionally harsh life caused much stress and ill health. Destiny must have chosen me to be there to help some of these desperate people. One night, about two months into my imprisonment - I had begun with six weeks in solitary confinement - that destiny revealed itself.

It was past 11 pm. I awakened to awareness of an inmate who was suffering excruciating stomach pain. He could not walk by himself. Two others were helping him stay upright. He was suffering from peptic ulcer disease and wanted medication. His face dropped when I told him I had not been allowed to bring medical supplies with me to the prison.

Then the breakthrough occurred!

I gave him two glasses of water.

His pain disappeared in minutes and he could begin to stand up by himself. He beamed from ear to ear. You cannot imagine the joy of relief he experienced, even in such harsh surroundings.

'What happens if the pain comes back?' he asked.

'Drink two glasses of water every three hours,' I replied.

He became pain-free and remained disease-free for the rest of his time in prison. His 'water cure' in that harsh environment amazed me as a doctor. I knew I had witnessed a healing power of water that I had not been taught in medical school. I felt sure that no similar observation had ever been made in medical research.

If water could cure a painful disease condition in such a stressful environment, surely it needed further research? I realised that my destiny as a healer had brought me to this 'human stress laboratory' to teach me a new approach to medicine and to reveal many other hidden secrets about the human body. I opened my eyes. Instinctively, I realised why I had ended up in prison!

I stopped thinking about myself and started to think about doing medical research. I began to identify the many health problems caused by the stress of prison. By far and away the largest number involved ulcer pains. I treated those who came to me with what proved to be the best natural 'elixir' - water. I found water could treat and cure more diseases than any other single medication I knew about.

It could even cure someone who was literally dying of pain! It was again past 11 pm. I was on my way to a sick inmate when I heard a piercing groan from a cell at the end of the corridor. I followed the sound and found a young man curled up on the floor of his cell. He seemed to be totally detached, giving out deep, piercing groans.

'What is wrong?' I asked.

He did not react. I had to shake him before he managed to reply, 'My ulcer is killing me.'

'What have you done for the pain?' I asked.

He haltingly explained, 'Since one o'clock ... when it started ... I have taken three Tagamets ... one full bottle of antacid ... but the pain has got worse since then.' (At that time, prisoners were able to get medications from the prison hospital.)

By now I had a much clearer understanding of peptic ulcer pain. What I did not realise until then was the severity it could reach, when not even strong medication could stop it. After examining his abdomen for possible complications, I gave him two glasses of tap water - just over one pint (0.5 litre). I left him to visit another sick inmate. Ten minutes later I returned. Groans of pain no longer filled the corridor.

'How do you feel?' I asked.

'Much better,' he replied, 'but I still have some pain.'

I gave him a third glass of water and his pain stopped completely within four minutes.

This man had been semi-conscious, on the verge of death. He had taken a huge amount of ulcer medication with no result. And now, after drinking only three glasses of tap water, he became pain-free, sitting up and socialising with friends.

What a humbling discovery. And I thought I had received the best medical education in the world, in London!

During nearly three years of my captivity, I cured over 3,000 ulcer cases with only water in Tehran's Evin Prison - 'my God-given stress laboratory'. All thanks to water. Plain, simple, cost-free medicine for everyone. Water that we all take for granted! Water that the medical profession has dismissed as unworthy of research!

Since my eyes were opened to water as a natural medication, I have developed and applied this technique to the point where it has alleviated and healed hundreds of traditionally incurable sicknesses and chronic pains. I have seen water completely reverse conditions such as asthma, angina, hypertension, migraine headaches, arthritis pain, back pain, colitis pain and chronic constipation, heartburn and hiatal hernia, depression, chronic fatigue syndrome, high cholesterol, morning sickness, overweight problems - even heart problems thought to need bypass surgery. All these disease conditions have responded simply and permanently to water. Ordinary, natural water.

This book reveals how water and salt can cure many health problems, by explaining what happens when there is not enough water in the body, and contains the information you need to apply this simple but effective discovery for your own well-being.

Where did modern medicine go wrong?

'If we doctors threw all our medicines into the sea, it would be that much better for our patients and that much worse for the fishes.'
- Oliver Wendell Holmes MD

The greatest tragedy in medical history in my opinion is the assumption that dry mouth is the only sign of the body's water needs. Based on this mistaken assumption, modern medicine has made confounding mistakes that have cost society dearly. Let us look at these four mistaken assumptions:

1. The whole structure of modern medicine is built on the flawed premise that *dry mouth is the only sign of dehydration.* This mistake is responsible for the lack of understanding about various painful health problems that result in premature death to many millions of people. They suffer because they do not know they are seriously thirsty. Modern, 'science-based' medicine is structured upon the simple dry mouth mistake that became established many years ago. In 1764, Albrecht von Haller, a German, first claimed dry mouth as a sign of thirst. In 1918, Walter Bradford Cannon, an English doctor, supported Haller's views. Since he was an influential person, these views became fashionable and are reflected in accepted scientific literature to this day.

Frenchman Moritz Schiff, however, had claimed in 1867 that thirst is a general sensation: 'It is no more a local sensation than hunger.' We now know that Haller and Cannon were wrong - but since theirs were the views that took root in the infrastructure of medicine, the same mistake has been passed on from one generation of medical students to another until the present day. This traditional flaw in the scientific understanding of the human body's water regulation altered the path of medicine. Schiff understood the human body better.

Actually, dry mouth is not a sign to rely on. The human body uses a different logic: to be able to chew and swallow food, and to facilitate and lubricate this function, ample saliva is produced even if the rest of the body is short of water. In any case, water is too important to the body to signal its shortage only through the experience of a dry mouth. The human body has many other sophisticated signals to indicate when it is short of water. The body can suffer from deep dehydration without showing a dry month. Dehydration produces severe symptoms, even to the point of causing life-threatening crises. Modern medicine has confused these symptoms of internal, localized droughts and has identified them as different diseases. As a result, toxic medications are prescribed to treat 'diseases' rather than the dehydration.

Dry mouth is one of the very last indicators of dehydration of the body. By the time dry mouth becomes an indicator of water shortage, many delicate functions of the body have been shut down and prepared for deletion. This is exactly how the ageing process is established - through a loss of enzyme functions. A dehydrated body loses sophistication and versatility. One example is juvenile diabetes, in which the insulin-producing cells of the pancreas are sacrificed as a result of persistent dehydration.

2. The second major mistake is the thinking *that water is a simple substance that only dissolves and circulates different things.* Water is not a simple, inert substance. It has two primary properties in the body. The first one is its life-sustaining properties. The other, more important role of water is its life-giving functions. Modern medicine recognizes only the life-sustaining properties of water. That is why chronic unintentional dehydration is ultimately an unrecognised life-threatening process. You need to recognize and understand the process to save your health and your life - naturally.

3. The third serious error in medicine is the premise that *the human body can efficiently regulate its water intake throughout the life of the person.* As we grow older, we lose our perception of thirst and fail to drink adequately, until the plum-like cells in vital

organs become prune-like and can no longer sustain life. We need to recognize the onset of dehydration and its manifestations to prevent the irreversible stages of the process.

4. The fourth nail in the coffin of present-day medicine is the thought that *any fluid can replace the water needs of the body*. This is a major problem at present. Some of the manufactured beverages in common use do not function in the body like natural water. If you begin to understand the natural reason some plants manufacture caffeine, or even cocaine, you will then recognize the problem. The information in this book is about one of the greatest of all health discoveries in the world, because it exposes an important tragedy in medical history - the erroneous assumption that the dry mouth state is the only sign of the body's water needs. Simply put, *the new scientific understanding is that chronic unintentional dehydration in the human body can manifest itself in as many ways as we in medicine have invented diseases.* We have created an opportunity for the drug industry to thrive, and have given birth to the current 'sick-care' health system at the expense of people's precious lives and resources. The sick-care system survives and thrives when people are continuously sick. This is exactly what is going on now.

Tragically, the medical breakthrough about dehydration as the origin of most health problems is not reaching the public through the commerce-directed health-maintenance systems in our countries. If it did, it would mean the rapid extinction of these systems. Yet there is no sane reason why tens of millions in our society should be medicated when all they suffer from is dehydration.

The statements in this chapter are not meant to reflect badly on the dedicated staff employed within the sick-care system, who daily render compassionate service to the unfortunate. They are not to be blamed for the fundamental mistakes in standard treatment protocols in medicine. The blame is directed at the medical professionals in powerful positions and the national health institutes that could correct the problem but have shown a reluctance to do so.

Mainstream medicine and its fund-raising sidekicks will not of their own accord abandon pharmaceutical medicine. Why? They do not want to allow *natural* solutions to the health problems of society to get clearance and reach the public. This book is designed to upset this self-serving trend, which benefits only the commercial healthcare systems in our advanced society to the detriment of the people. It is now crystal clear that the human body has many different ways of showing its general or local water needs. These manifestations of drought in the body have been assumed to be indicators of this or that disease condition. Based on this ignorance, and protected and coddled by the pharmaceutical industry, mainstream medicine has labelled the different complications of dehydration as various 'diseases'. On the basis of this erroneous assumption, the trusting American public has to pay ever-increasing healthcare costs with their health and hard-earned money.

We must understand that persistent dehydration brings about a continuously changing new chemical state in the body. When a new dehydration-produced chemical state becomes fully established, it causes many structural changes, even to the genetic blueprints of the body. This is why prevention of dehydration is crucial. This is also why childhood asthma is a major health issue with me, as is non-infectious earache in infants. Dehydration, to the point of causing asthma in children, can ultimately cause genetic damage, autoimmune diseases and even cancer in their later years. Understanding chronic dehydration will clear the way for the development of an infinitely more people-friendly healthcare system. It will be possible, in my estimation, to have a decidedly healthier and productive nation at 30 per cent of the present healthcare costs. As you see, I am not promoting a moneymaking product. I am only sharing a unique medical insight and the outcome of my many years of research that

15

will help medical professionals and the public understand the basic cause of so many conditions of ill-health.

We are in the twenty-first century, yet even at this stage of our development, the outward manifestations of regional dehydration have not been understood by us in medicine. We have always looked for a drug solution to throw at a health concern. We have not succeeded at limiting these health concerns; rather, we have constantly expanded the list and thrown more drugs at them. We have truly caused a costly chaos in the name of modern medicine with no end in sight. We now have significant problems that beg urgent solutions. As Albert Einstein observed: *'The significant problems we have cannot be solved at the same level of thinking with which we created them.'* We obviously need a new approach to medical science to solve our health problems.

The solution to the present human-made and drug-industry-protected health concerns of society can only be physiology-based. Understanding the molecular physiology of dehydration will restructure the future practice of clinical medicine. It will cause *a fundamental paradigm change* in the science of medicine. By showing the way to enhance the natural healing powers of the body within the discipline of physiology, the pharmaceutical approach to our present health problems will be completely replaced. The primary focus in medicine will become *disease prevention* rather than its protracted, cost-intensive and invasive treatment protocols.

Water – the 'new' science

'A new scientific truth is not usually presented in a way to convince its opponents. Rather, they die off and a rising generation is familiarized with the truth from the start.' **- Max Planck**

Phillip Day: Amazingly, few meaningful studies have been carried out on the metabolic effects of water on the human body, let alone its biophysical properties. In April 2008, a study from the University of Pennsylvania concluded that, from the perusal of existing scientific literature, drinking water had no special benefits beyond flushing toxins from the kidneys. The media took this to mean, 'carry on drinking tea, coffee and sodas, and get all the water you need from those!' But what the researchers actually said was, *'Although we wish we could demolish all of the urban myths found on the Internet regarding the benefits of supplemental water ingestion, we concede there is also no clear evidence of lack of benefit. In fact, there is simply a lack of evidence in general.'*[4]

In other words, water has not been studied in relation to human health, even though the body is approximately 73% water, the brain 85% water, and the planet we inhabit 73% water and salt solution. Even more bizarre is the fact that water has already been confirmed by Japanese scientist Dr Masaru Emoto and others to be a reactor to sophisticated information, yet the Descartian, matter-only approach of science remains in denial.

The work of Drs Bruce Lipton, Rupert Sheldrake, Cleve Backster, Professor William Tiller and others point categorically to 'matter as energy', and how our thoughts, emanating from a water-predominant brain, directly affect matter.[5] Medicine acknowledges this as the

---

[4] http://news.bbc.co.uk/2/hi/health/7326437.stm

[5] Lipton, Bruce, *The Biology of Belief*, Elite Books, 2005; Tiller, Dibble et al, *Conscious Acts of Creation, the Emergence of a New Physics*, Pavior, 2001

placebo effect but declines to enquire further. There is no bedside manner. There is no money to be made out of thoughts or good feelings. Yet history reveals an astonishing perspective with water. For centuries, water-dowsing has been used to find water for wells. Romans set up baths and wells and swore by their healing properties. Lourdes and other religious sites boast 'healing' waters with unusual biophysical properties. The Bible, Koran and other religious writings contain many references to water which are hardly anecdotal. Water washes sins away as well as dirt. In the New Testament, Jesus, John and the Apostles all baptised with water: *'Most assuredly I say to you, unless one is born of water and the Spirit, he cannot enter the kingdom of God.'*[6] Evidently the ancients knew water transcended its physical constraints and was indeed 'sacred'. Today, scientists are still baffled by its biochemical uniqueness, as Peter Ferreira and Dr Barbara Hendel point out in their *Water and Salt, The Essence of Life:*

'The formula, H_2O, defines water chemically but it doesn't say anything about its inherent nature. From a biochemical and biophysical point of view, water is an anomaly because it behaves in ways that scientists don't expect it to. The boiling point of water, according to physical law, should be as low as 114.8°F. However, it boils at 212°F. When water freezes and becomes solid, it expands instead of contracting in volume, as would be expected. At 98.6°F, which is our body's normal temperature, water has its lowest specific heat. At this temperature the greatest amount of energy is needed to effect a change in the temperature. This abnormal physical behaviour of water plays a central role in life on Earth, because, in fact, it enables the existence of life. If water would only behave "normally" in one aspect, there would be no life on Earth.'[7]

Dr Batmanghelidj: The new scientific truth and level of thinking about the human body that will empower people to become

---

[6] John 3:5 NKJV
[7] **Hendel Dr B and P Ferreira,** *Water and Salt – The Essence of Life,* 2003

practitioners of preventive medicine for themselves is as follows: <u>It is the solvent—the water content—that regulates all functions of the body, including the activity of all the solutes (the solids) that are dissolved in it.</u> The disturbances in water metabolism of the body (the solvent metabolism) produce a variety of signals, indicating a 'system' disturbance in the particular functions associated with the water supply and its rationed regulation.

Let me repeat, <u>every function of the body is monitored and pegged to the efficient flow of water.</u> 'Water distribution' is the only way of making sure that not only an adequate amount of water but its transported elements – hormones, chemical messengers and nutrients – first reach the more vital organs. In turn, every organ that produces a substance to be made available to the rest of the body will only monitor its own rate and standards of production and release into the flowing water according to constantly changing quotas that are set by the brain. Once the water itself reaches the 'drier' areas, it also exercises its many other most vital and missing physical and chemical regulatory actions.

Within this view, water intake and its priority distribution achieve paramount importance. The regulating neurotransmitter systems (histamine and its subordinate agents) become increasingly active during the regulation of water requirements of the body. Their action should not be continuously blocked by the use of medication. Their purpose should be understood and satisfied by drinking more water. I have made exactly the same statements to a body of scientists that had gathered from all over the world in Monte Carlo in 1989 for a conference on the topic of inflammation, analgesics and immune modulators.

The new paradigm permits an incorporation of the 'fourth dimension of time' into scientific research [consistency]. It will facilitate an understanding of the damaging effect of an establishing dehydration that persists and continues to increase *during any duration of time*. It will make it possible to forecast the physiological events that will lead to disease states in the future, including what at present appear as genetic disorders. It will transform the present 'shot in the dark, symptom-based' approach to the practice of medicine into a scientifically accurate medical art; it will make preventive forecasting possible. It will establish excellent health and reduce healthcare costs to individuals and to any society that fosters its spread.

However, since water shortage in different areas of the body will manifest varying symptoms, signals and complications now labelled as diseases, as soon as water is offered as a natural solution, people may think this could not be so! Water cures so many diseases? No way!

Speaking thus, they shut their minds to the new possibility of preventing and possibly even curing so many different 'dis-eases' that are dehydration-produced. It does not occur to them that the only remedy for conditions that come about when the body begins to get dehydrated is water and nothing else. A number of sample testimonials are published at the end of this book to open sceptical eyes to the fact that the greatest health discovery of all times <u>is that water is a natural medication for a variety of health conditions</u>.

Water regulation at different stages of life

There are basically three stages to water regulation of the body in the different phases of life. One, the stage of life of a foetus in the uterus of the mother. Two, the phase of growth until full height and width is achieved (between the ages of 18 to 25). Three, the phase of life from fully grown stage to the demise of the person.

During the intrauterine stage of cell expansion, water for cell growth of the child has to be provided by the mother. However, the transmitter system for water intake seems to be produced by the foetal tissue but registers its effect on the mother. The very first indicator for water needs of the foetus and the mother seems to be the early morning sickness during the early phase of pregnancy. The early morning sickness of the mother is a thirst signal of both the foetus and the mother.

It is now becoming obvious that because of a gradually failing thirst sensation, the body becomes chronically and increasingly dehydrated from an early adult age. With increase in age, the water content of the cells of the body decreases to the point that the ratio of the volume of body water that is inside the cells to that which is outside the cells changes from a figure of 1.1 to almost 0.8. This is a very drastic change. Since the water that we drink provides for the cell function and volume requirements, the decrease in our daily water intake affects the efficiency of cell activity. As a result, chronic dehydration causes symptoms of disease when the variety of emergency signals of dehydration are not understood—as they are until now not understood. These urgent cries of the body for water are treated as abnormal and dealt with by the use of medications.

The human body can become dehydrated even when abundant water is readily available. Humans seem to lose their thirst sensation and the critical perception of needing water. Not recognizing their water need, they become gradually, increasingly and chronically dehydrated with the progress in age. Further confusion lies in the idea that when the sensation of thirst urges us, tea, coffee, or alcohol-containing beverages can be taken as a substitute.

As already stated, the 'dry mouth' is the very last sign of dehydration. The body can suffer from dehydration even when the mouth may be fairly moist. Still worse, in the elderly, the mouth can be seen to be obviously dry and yet thirst may not be acknowledged and satisfied.

Water has other important properties

Scientific research shows that water has many other properties besides being a solvent and means of transport. Not having paid attention to the other properties of water in the regulation of different functions in the body has produced pitiful confusions in our so-called science-based modern medicine. Water has two classical roles for all living matter: Life-giving properties and life-sustaining properties.

Some life-giving properties:

1) Water has a firmly established and essential hydrolytic role in all aspects of body metabolism: water-dependent chemical reactions (hydrolysis). This property of water 'drives all chemical reactions' that 'create life'. Water is the source of energy for the creation of life. **Six hundred units of energy becomes over five thousand units after hydrolysis so that life can move into the space of time and go forward.**[8]

2) At the cell membrane, the osmotic flow of water can also generate 'hydroelectric' energy (voltage gradient) that is stored in the energy pools in form of ATP (adenosine triphosphate) and GTP (guanosine triphosphate) and used for elemental (cation) exchanges, particularly in neurotransmission. ATP is a chemical source of energy in the body, so is GTP. The energy generated by water helps manufacture ATP and GTP. This property of water makes it possible for life to 'blossom' and become animated.

3) Water also forms a particular structure pattern and shape that seems to be employed as the adhesive material in the bondage of the cell architecture. Like glue, it sticks the solid structures in the cell membrane together. It develops the stickiness of 'ice' at higher body temperatures. This property of water makes it possible for life to regenerate itself on the DNA assembly line in a series of 'protected'

---

[8] **Batmanghelidj, F,** *Your Body's Many Cries For Water,* Tagman Press, 2000

and walled environments — thoroughly protected environments within other environments.

Some life-sustaining properties

Water is a solvent. Water is a means of transport. Water is a packing material. These properties of water make it possible for *life to survive and exist* within a 'life-span' in the society of other life-forms. Some of what water does is as follows:

- The proteins and enzymes of the body function more efficiently in solutions of lower viscosity; this is true of all the receptors in the cell membranes — means of command and control message system
- In solutions of higher viscosity (in a dehydrated state) the proteins and enzymes become less efficient
- Recognition of thirst of the body becomes less accurate as the body becomes increasingly dehydrated in the interior of cells — the process of aging
- Water itself regulates all functions of the body, including the activity of solutes it carries

The new paradigm — "Water, the solvent of the body, regulates all functions, including the activity of the solutes it dissolves and circulates" — should become the basis of all future approach to medical research. Thus, histamine formation and release is a function that is directly connected to the concentration and viscosity of the internal solutions in the body. Histamine becomes engaged in order to correct the concentration imbalance produced by dehydration. One of the most vital responsibilities of histamine in maintaining concentration balance is exercised in the central nervous system and its vast network of nerves and their distribution throughout the body.

The products manufactured in the brain cells are transported to their destination within the nerves in different parts of the body on 'waterways'. Nerve cells are said to be 85 percent water. And there seems to exist small waterways or micro-streams along the length of nerves that 'float' the packaged materials along 'guidelines', known as microtubules. These products are taken to the nerve endings of their respective cells for use in the brain's communication system in the entire body.

When the body is dehydrated, a 'locked-in' drive for water intake, as well as a rationing and distribution system for the available water according to a predetermined priority program, becomes established throughout the body—a form of drought management. It should be remembered that the body does not have a reserve of water to draw on; it operates a priority distribution system for the amount of water available from intake.

It has become scientifically clear that a histamine-directed and -operated neurotransmitter system becomes active and initiates the subordinate systems that ration available water. At the same time, these processes promote the intake of new water by initiating the thirst signals of the body. They also redistribute, according to a preset priority, the amount of water that is in circulation, or can be drawn away from other areas.

The subordinate systems employ as their intermediary agents:
- Vasopressin (vayso-press-in),
- Renin-angiotensin (RA),
- Prostaglandins (prosta-glan-din, PG)
- Kinins (ky-nin)

In the amphibian species, it has been shown that histamine reserves and their rate of generation are at minimal levels. In the same species, histamine generation becomes established and gets pronounced whenever the animal is dehydrated.

A proportionate increase in the production rate and storage of the neurotransmitter histamine for rationing regulation of the available water in dehydrated animals—drought management—becomes established. Histamine and its subordinate water-intake and distribution regulators – prostaglandins, kinins, and PAF (another histamine-associated agent) – also cause pain when they come across pain-sensing nerves in the body.

The above "view shift" in medical science establishes two major points that have been disregarded until now:

- One, the body can become dehydrated as we age. At the same time, it discards 'dry mouth' as the only indicator of body thirst.
- Two, when histamine and its subordinate water regulators become excessively active—to the point of causing allergies, asthma, chronic pains and other manifestations in different parts of the body – these symptoms and pains should be translated as one of a variety of crisis signals of water shortage in the body—an emergency thirst signal.

This 'paradigm shift' will now make it possible to recognize many diverse, associated signals of general or local body dehydration and label them for what they are—not diseases but simply states of dehydration.

Pain: Cries of thirst

The adoption of this paradigm shift dictates that chronic pains of the body that cannot be explained as injury or infection should first and foremost be interpreted as signals of chronic water shortage in the area where pain is registered—a *local thirst*. These pain signals should be considered and excluded as primary indicators for dehydration of the body before any other complicated procedures are forced on the patient. Non-infectious, 'recurring' or chronic pains should be viewed as indicators of body thirst.

Pain is a sensation that denotes local chemical changes in the area around the nerves that monitor the acid/alkali balance. The mechanism is designed to safeguard against a build-up of excess acid from metabolism that 'could burn' and eat into the cell membranes and inner structures of cells. When water has not been available to wash the acidic toxic waste of metabolism, the nerve endings sense the change and report it to the brain's pain centres. Up to a point, the brain suppresses the sensation to let the corrective processes deal with the problem. There comes a time, however, that the conscious mind must be warned of the water shortage. When the significance of pain as an emergency thirst signal is not recognized, the intensity of pain increases until movement and mobility of the area are affected—to prevent the production of additional toxic waste.

Not recognizing the phenomenon of pain for what it is—a sophisticated localized thirst signal of the body—will undoubtedly produce complicated problems. It is all too easy to assume these signals are complications of serious disease processes and to treat dehydration with toxic chemicals and complicated procedures. Even though water by itself will alleviate the condition, medications or invasive diagnostic procedures may still be forced on the person. It is the responsibility of both patients and their doctors to be aware of the damage chronic dehydration can cause in the human body.

The pains of dehydration and their medical labels include:
- Dyspeptic pain
- Rheumatoid arthritis pain
- Anginal pain (heart pain on walking or even at rest)
- Low back pain
- Intermittent claudication pain (leg pain on walking)
- Migraine and hangover headaches

- Colitis pain and its associated constipation
- False appendicitis pain

Dehydration and some chronic pains

This new scientific perspective dictates that all these pains should be treated with a regular adjustment to daily water intake. No less than two and a half quarts (two and one half litres) in 24 hours should be taken for a few days prior to the routine and regular use of analgesics or other pain-relieving medications such as antihistamine or antacids — well before permanent local or general damage can establish and reach an irreversible disease status. If the problem has persisted for many years, those who wish to test the pain-relieving property of water should make sure their kidneys can make sufficient urine so that they do not retain too much water in the body. Urine output should be measured against water intake. With increase in water intake, the urine output should also increase.

This new perspective of the mechanism of pain production in dehydration will shed light on complicated disease conditions in future research. It exposes the long-term use of analgesics for silencing a cardinal signal of chronic and localized dehydration in the above classical 'diseases' as detrimental to the well-being of the body.

In their own right, analgesics can cause fatal side-effects, apart from the damage caused by the ongoing dehydration temporarily silenced without removing the root cause of these pains — dehydration! Very often, these analgesics cause gastrointestinal bleeding. A few thousand people die every year from this complication. It is clear that over-the-counter painkillers can cause liver and kidney damage also in some users.

The scientific background for the above views, covered in my other books, is also available to scientists in pain research. This book is intended to brush aside the professional resistance of the AMA and

NIH, which are aware of my findings and have, contrary to their oath and obligations to society, refused to propagate it to the benefit of the public. The new discovery of the role of water in the body can work wonders in the future practice of clinical medicine. That is why these professional bodies, who gain financially by promulgating their 'Dark Ages' philosophy, have not engaged in research of the information about complications associated with lack of sufficient water in the human body.

The moment the medical professionals adopt this paradigm shift, the present form of 'ignorance of the human body based medical practice' will transform to a thoughtful, preventive approach to healthcare. More importantly, simple physiology-based cures to early disease emergence will become available, well before irreversible pathology can become established.

Hydroelectric energy

"The desire to take medicine is perhaps the greatest feature which distinguishes man from animals." - **William Osler**

Phillip Day: The discovery that water is an information system is a very exciting development. Professor William Tiller et al report:

Ice Crystal Patterns Materialize Specific Intentions in Water: In his recent book, 'The Message From Water', Dr Masaru Emoto has shown that, under what appeared to be well controlled conditions, ice crystal formation in water appears to display relatively unique patterns dependent, not only on the chemical toxicity of various lakes, springs, glaciers and cities where the water is collected, which is to be expected, but also upon (1) specific music played in a precise environment, (2) wrapping printed statements of appreciation, thanks, anger, hate, etc. on the jars of this water for a given time, (3) specific subtle energies (chi, hado) expressed in the water environment and (4) specific essence additions to water. In all of these examples, it is difficult to evaluate the proportion of the effect on ice crystal pattern formation that comes directly from the physical factors involved and the portion that comes indirectly from the held intentions of the humans involved in the process. It is our belief that a meaningful portion of these beautiful ice crystal patterns arise indirectly from the latter and this provides a perfect stage for us to now describe the details of our own experiments on water.

Hendel and Ferreira point out that each snow crystal is unique, yet when melted and then reformed at 23°C, the same crystal is formed:

'Every water molecule has its own unmistakable identity. It is energy that forms matter, not the other way around! Water is more than simply H₂O. Work in the field of photon research has revealed remarkable discoveries. It takes more than one billion light quanta to build only one single water molecule. This complements the discoveries of the Swiss atomic physicist and

29

Nobel Prize winner, Dr. Carlo Rubbia. He was able to demonstrate, through a mathematical ratio, that it takes more than one billion energy units in order to manifest a single unit of matter. Photons are pure light energy. They align each and every single water molecule in their own unique way and give each its unmistakable identity (exactly as for human beings and all other life forms).

If we apply this information to our physical body, this insight suggests that organs in our body can only change when the energy that manifests, and is continuously supporting the manifestation of the organ, changes. If this change demands an energy deficit, we become ill. However, if we give our body the correct information, it will be able to heal itself again.'[9]

How would you like to find the seat of that intelligence? More to the point, can we afford to ignore the properties of water science has yet to explain?

Dr Batmanghelidj: If eating is about providing energy for the human body, *water is more important as a source of energy than anything else we eat.* This is where confusion has arisen in the application of science to human behaviour. All our health problems stem from the misconception that food is the only source of energy to the human body. We speak of the hydrolysis of this or that element in the body – the term refers to the breakdown of a substance through the action of water – yet we have never realized that the chemical processes <u>involve the transfer of energy from water to whatever is being broken down</u>.

As previously mentioned, Scientists George and Associates have studied the formula for energy transfer from water and have shown that hydrolysis adds one zero – increases by one order of magnitude – to the energy content of a substance in the process of breaking it down. It's a bit like dripping oil on top of a piece of wood that has a hard

---

9 Hendel and Ferreira, op. cit.

time burning. You stimulate the burning process and get a more intense fire. In the body, chemical reactions become more intense when water is available. George *et al.* have shown that the energy content in a standard weight of magnesium-ATP, which is 600 Joule units before it is broken down, becomes 5,850 Joule units when it is hydrolyzed. Thus, as I see it, the chemical reactions that constantly take place in our bodies because of the action of water energize the body by one order of magnitude.

Taking this newly understood effect of hydrolysis to its logical conclusion, a total re-evaluation of our understanding of the human metabolism becomes unavoidable. For example, if one egg possesses about 70 calories, when the body begins to hydrolyze and metabolize the components of the egg, the output of energy from its metabolism may reach about 700 calories. Not having taken into consideration the energizing effect of water in the chemical reactions of the body, the traditional evaluation of the energy consumption of the body for its myriad chemical reactions suffers from inaccuracy and underestimation. *This is why we have failed to consider the need to hydrate the body before any food intake* - hence the many unsolved health problems in modern medical science.

Now you know water is the primary source of energy in all chemical reactions associated with food metabolism of the body, you now understand the wisdom of making water available to prepare the body for food processing. Food is similar to fossil fuel in traditional power plants; it is 'dirty' energy and has much residue. The outcome of relying more on food as the primary source of energy is disease: obesity, cholesterol deposits, diabetes, hypertension, depression, neurological disorders such as multiple sclerosis, Alzheimer's disease, various cancers, and many, many more.

Hydroelectricity: the preferred source of energy for all body functions

Water has yet another infinitely more important role in energy formation in the body. It is responsible for the manufacture of hydroelectricity, primarily for the functions of the brain. This form of energy is 'clean' - it has almost no residue or waste products. Excess water is excreted in the form of urine. It does not stay in the body in a 'lake' the way excess food forms mountains of fat. The hydroelectric form of energy is much more suited to the delicate metabolism of the brain.

It is uncanny the way water is used to make electricity inside the cells to energize the intricate functions that keep the cells alive and productive. Certain proteins are found within the membranes of every cell in the body. These proteins have an affinity for certain minerals available in the blood circulation and the solution surrounding the cells. Some of these proteins collect sodium and potassium, some magnesium, and some calcium. These minerals, when attached to their specific protein, get spun by the rush of water and begin to shift with the fast rotation of the protein. This process manufactures electricity that gets stored in the membrane stockpiles known as ATP or GTP (guanosine triphosphate). In this energy-generating process, the appropriate minerals are also relocated to balance the osmotic ratio between the outside and inside of the cells. Philippa M Wiggin has described the fundamentals of this process as follows:

The mechanism that controls or brings about the effective function of the cation pumps utilizes the energy-transforming property of water, the solvent: *"The source of energy for cation transport or ATP synthesis lies in increases in chemical potentials with increasing hydration of small cations and polyphosphate anions in the highly structured interfacial aqueous phase of the two phosphorylated intermediates."* Waiting to get thirsty, when the body fluids become concentrated before thirst is induced, one loses the energy-generating properties of water in the dehydrated cells of the body. This is the major reason why we should prevent dehydration rather than wait to correct it. This new understanding of the role of water in cation exchange is enough justification for letting the body engage in prudent surplus water management rather than forcing it into drought water management.[10]

The fact that *the interior* of the body's cells becomes drastically dehydrated when the body is short of water is the most important phenomenon to understand. In dehydration, 66 per cent of the water loss is from the interior of the cells, 26 per cent of the loss is from extracellular fluid volume, and only 8 per cent is borne by the blood tissue in the vascular system, which constricts within its network of capillaries and maintains the integrity of the circulation system. Thus, dehydrated cells begin to run low on energy reserves and start to suffer. They begin to reflect their dehydration by producing various symptoms of inefficient performance in the routine functions of the body. The brain is the most vulnerable organ of the body to this problem.

There are about nine trillion brain and nerve cells in the body. They constantly communicate with one another to keep the body in sync with its environment. As it happens, the best and preferred source of clean energy they use for these complicated activities is hydroelectric energy. This is the reason a glass of water is the best pick-me-up. It will energize the brain out of its listlessness in a matter of minutes. If you were to tap into the energy of food for this purpose, not only would you need water to digest the food for its eventual use, but the process would take quite a time. First the food is converted to sugar, and then the sugar is used by the brain cells as a source of energy.

---

[10] Wiggins PM, 'A Mechanism of ATP-Driven Cation Pumps'; *Biophysics of Water*, John Wiley and Sons, Ltd. 1982

The human brain is roughly 1/50 of the total body weight. The brain cells are said to be 85 per cent water. Twenty per cent of blood circulation is allocated and made available to the brain. This means the brain gets to pick and choose from the circulating blood what is needed for its normal functions. The brain puts the body to sleep but does not shut itself off at night. It works all the time, running the heart, lungs, liver, the glands, blood circulation and so on. It processes all the information from different parts of the body as well as whatever enters it from daily exposure to the physical, social and electromagnetic environment.

To process all these inputs and alert all parts of the body for a coordinated response, the brain expends a vast quantity of energy. At the same time, it expends energy in manufacturing the primary chemical messengers (neurotransmitters), which must then be transported to nerve endings. The transportation system also uses a vast quantity of energy. This high rate of energy consumption by the brain is, in my opinion, the main reason it receives about 20 per cent of blood circulation. It needs the water the blood tissue contains to make hydroelectricity. Naturally, water will also deliver the pick of the raw materials the brain needs to manufacture its chemicals.

There is a threshold for energy release for some inputs. The brain calculates and understands what is important and what is not for its energy expenditure. When ATP reserves are low, many stimuli do not invoke a response. This low ATP reserve in some overactive brain cells will become reflected as a fatigue state in the functions that are controlled by those brain cells. This is why food is not a good immediate pick-me-up but water is.

The central control system in the brain happens to recognize the low energy levels available for its functions. The sensations of thirst or hunger also stem from low, ready-to-access energy levels. To mobilize energy from what is stored in the fat, hormonal release mechanisms are needed. This takes a while longer (and requires some physical activity for energy release) than the urgent needs of the brain. The front of the brain gets energy either from hydroelectricity or from sugar in blood circulation. The brain's need for water is constant and urgent:

- One, to form hydroelectric energy for message transmission
- Two, because the transport systems across the cell membranes of the brain depend on adequate water. The membrane barriers need to be more 'fluid' to facilitate transport of materials from blood to brain
- Three, because the energy from hydroelectricity is also needed for all transport systems in the 'water channels' within the nerves that connect the brain to different parts of the body

These are the three main reasons why brain tissue is 85 per cent water and is almost always thirsty. If you confuse this brain thirst for hunger just because the sensations are similar, you will create a physiological state conducive to premature ageing, disease, decay and early death. Obesity, depression, and cancer are three of the labels we in medicine have created to describe the killer process of persistent unintentional dehydration in the human body.

In a dehydrated state, the human body begins initially to inhibit some functions but will eventually dismantle its structures and components. As an example, consider the two forms of diabetes. In type II diabetes, insulin production and release is inhibited. In type I diabetes the insulin-producing beta-cells are destroyed from inside. Both forms of diabetes are the direct consequence of unintentional dehydration – or more pertinently, medical ignorance about the importance of water to health and well-being. The body has no alternative but to deal strictly and economically with problems of dehydration. Thus, there is a metabolic component to dehydration we must understand to reverse a disease process. When I use the word

35

dehydration, I am not referring to water shortage only. I am also speaking of the shortage of any raw materials that culminates in a disease state.

Salt

'Your table salt is actually 97.5% sodium chloride and 2.5% chemicals such as moisture absorbents and iodine. Dried at over 1,200 degrees Fahrenheit, the excessive heat alters the natural chemical structure of the salt causing the potential for a myriad of health problems in your body.' – **Dr Joseph Mercola**

'...all of us have in our veins the exact same percentage of salt in our blood that exists in the ocean, and, therefore, we have salt in our blood, in our sweat, in our tears. We are tied to the ocean.'
– John F Kennedy

Phillip Day: Before we examine Dr B's work on various disease conditions and their associations with dehydration, let us consider salt.

Salt consumption for health is considered by the orthodoxy to be 'irresponsible' and 'dangerous', yet, so far as proper research has shown, the only danger to the public lies in *common table salt*, an industrial poison, which has been refined from Nature's storehouse to remove all elements but sodium chloride, then fortified with iodine and various fillers for the supermarket shelves. Some say we ended up with this particular compound due to industry's colossal use of it. Whatever the reason, *table salt is not real 'salt'* as the ancients knew it and its dangers are well touted:

- It destabilises blood pressure
- Can cause cellulite, kidney stones and rheumatism
- Upsets your fluid balance
- Acts as a diuretic (expels water from cells)
- Thereby a cell-toxin
- Contains the endocrine disrupters, fluoride and iodine
- Contains fillers such as calcium carbonate and aluminium hydroxide, the latter aluminium implicated in Alzheimer's Disease

Some PR job to convince the world we need it! Yet, as we're about to find out, 'salt' is essential for the body's systems. Farmers know if they don't put out the salt licks for their cattle, they die. This is real salt as Nature intended, not the truncated, worse-than-useless mess made of it in the refining process.

Enter saltpan salt, sea salt, Celtic salt, and the pink Dalek of all salts, Himalayan crystallized salt, or 'white gold' as it's come to be known (light pink gold, actually). Far from being the over-hyped, 'luxury' salt scorned by the media, leading Internet physician, Dr Joseph Mercola, declares that this mother-of-all-salts:

- *Regulates the water content throughout your body*
- *Balances excess acidity from your cells, particularly your brain cells*
- *Balances your blood sugar levels and helps reduce your aging rate*
- *Assists in the generation of hydroelectric energy in cells in your body and absorption of food particles through your intestinal tract*
- *Helps clear mucus plugs and phlegm from your lungs - particularly useful in asthma and cystic fibrosis*
- *Acts as a strong natural antihistamine to help clear up congestion in your sinuses*
- *Prevents muscle cramps*
- *Makes the structure of your bones firm - osteoporosis can occur when your body needs more salt and takes it from your bones*
- *Regulates your sleep - it is a natural hypnotic*
- *Maintains your libido*
- *Prevents varicose veins and spider veins on your legs and thighs*
- *Stabilizes irregular heartbeats - in conjunction with water, [salt] is actually essential for the regulation of blood pressure*[11]

Sea salt is sometimes used by those who wish to safeguard their health. The problem is, while sea salt is heavily mineralised, it can also

---

[11] www.mercola.com

contain industrial poisons cast into the oceans over the years. For that reason more pristine salts are often preferred – hence today's preference for the Himalayan variety.

Salt of the Ancients

Hendel and Ferreira write: *'Upon close examination, we find that the human body is made primarily of water and salt. Natural crystal salt contains all the elements of which the human body is comprised.*

...Our ancestors were already aware of the crucial necessity of salt. Wherever they found salt they guarded it like a treasure. Later in history, salt was called white gold and was the subject of political power plays, which oftentimes resulted in war. Roman soldiers were actually paid with salt, which is reflected in the word 'salary'. Salt was more important for survival than gold.'[12]

Online encyclopaedia, Wikipedia.org, records: *'There are thirty-five verses which reference salt in the English translation of the Bible (King James Version), the earliest being the story of Lot's wife, who was turned into a pillar of salt when she disobediently looked back at the wicked city of Sodom (Genesis 19:26). When King Abimelech destroyed the city of Shechem he is said to have 'sowed salt on it', a phrase expressing the completeness of its ruin (Judges 9:45). In the Sermon on the Mount, Jesus referred to his followers as the 'salt of the earth'. The apostle Paul also encouraged Christians to 'let your conversation be always full of grace, seasoned with salt' (Colossians 4:6).*

Salt is mandatory in the rite of the Tridentine Mass. Salt is used in the third item (which includes an Exorcism) of the Celtic Consecration (cf. Gallican rite) that is employed in the consecration of a church. Salt may be added to the water 'where it is customary' in the Roman Catholic rite of Holy Water. In the native Japanese religion Shinto, salt is used for ritual

---

[12] Hendel and Ferreira, op. cit.

purification of locations and people, such as in Sumo Wrestling. In Aztec mythology, Huixtocihuatl was a fertility goddess who presided over salt and salt water.'

Dr Batmanghelidj: Salt is a vital substance for the survival of all living creatures, particularly humans, and especially people with asthma, allergies and autoimmune disease.

Salt is a 'medication' that has been used by healers throughout the ages. In certain cultures, it is worth its weight in gold and is, in fact, exchanged weight for weight for gold. In desert countries, people know that salt intake is their insurance for survival. To these people, salt mines are synonymous with gold mines.

After many years of salt being bad-mouthed by ignorant health professionals and their media parrots, the importance of salt as a dietary supplement is once again being acknowledged and recognized. I was one of the early voices bringing about this change.

Water, salt and potassium together regulate the water content of the body. Water regulates the water content of the interior of the cell by working its way into all the cells it reaches. It has to get there to cleanse and extract the toxic waste of cell metabolism. Once water gets into the cells, the potassium content of the cells holds on to it and keeps it there - to the extent that potassium is available inside the cells. Even in the plant kingdom, it is potassium in the fruit that gives it firmness by holding water in the interior of the fruit. Our daily food contains ample potassium from its natural sources of fruits and vegetables, but not salt from its natural source. That is why we need to add salt to our daily diet. (Note: do not take too much potassium as a dietary supplement. It could cause trouble). Salt forces some water to keep it company outside the cells (osmotic retention of water by salt). It balances the amount of water that is held outside the cells.

Basically, there are two oceans of water in the body: one is held inside the cells of the body and the other held outside. Good health depends on a most delicate balance between the volumes of these two oceans. This balance is achieved by the regular intake of water, potassium-rich fruits and vegetables that also contain the vitamins needed by the body, and salt. Unrefined sea salt, which contains some of the other minerals that the body needs, is preferable. Sea salt may not contain enough iodine to keep the thyroid gland working normally, and it may enlarge into a goitre. Regular intake of a multivitamin that contains iodine is essential. Another source of iodine is dried kelp capsules, which are available from vitamin shops.

When water is not available to get into the cells freely, it is filtered from the outside salty ocean and injected into cells that are being overworked despite their water shortage. This secondary and emergency means of supplying important cells with injected water is the reason, in severe dehydration, that we retain salt and develop oedema [swelling] - to have more water available to draw from for filtration and injection into the cells.

The design of our bodies is such that the extent of the ocean of water outside the cells is expanded to have extra water in reserve for filtration and emergency injection into vital cells. To achieve this, the brain commands an increase in salt and water retention by the kidneys. This directive of the brain is the reason we get oedema when we don't drink enough water.

When water shortage in the body reaches a more critical level, and delivery of water by its injection into the cells becomes the main route of supply to more and more cells, an associated rise in injection pressure becomes necessary. The significant rise in pressure needed to inject water into the cells becomes measurable and is labelled 'hypertension', or high blood pressure.

Initially, the process of water filtration and its delivery into the cells is more efficient at night when the body is horizontal. In this position, the collected water, which settles mostly in the legs during the day, does not have to fight the force of gravity to get into the blood circulation. If reliance on this process of emergency hydration of some cells continues for long, the lungs begin to get waterlogged at night, and breathing becomes difficult. The person needs more pillows to sit upright to sleep. This condition is called cardiac asthma, and it is the consequence of dehydration. However, in this condition you must not overload the system by drinking too much water at the beginning. Increases in water intake must be slow and spaced out until urine production begins to increase at the same rate that you drink water. When we drink enough water to pass clear urine, we also pass out a lot of the salt that was held back. This is how we can get rid of oedema fluid from the body. Not by diuretics but by more water! Water is the best natural diuretic that exists.

In a person who has extensive oedema and whose heart sometimes beats irregularly or rapidly with little effort, the increase in water intake should be gradual and spaced out but water should not be withheld from the body. Salt intake should be limited for two or three days because the body is still in an overdrive mode to retain it. Once the oedema has cleared, salt should again be added to the diet. If there are irregular heartbeats, or the pulse is fast and furious but there is no oedema, increased water, salt, and other minerals such as magnesium, calcium, and some potassium will alleviate the problem.

Salt has many other functions than just regulating the water content of the body. Here are some of its additional duties:

- Salt is a strong, natural antihistamine. It can be used to relieve asthma by putting it on the tongue after drinking a glass or two of water. It is as effective as an inhaler, without the toxicity. You should drink one or two glasses of water before putting salt on the tongue

- Salt is a strong 'anti-stress' element for the body
- Salt is vital for extracting excess acidity from inside the cells, particularly the brain cells. If you don't want Alzheimer's disease, don't go salt-free, and don't let *them* put you on diuretic medications for long!
- Salt is vital for the kidneys to clear excess acidity and pass the acidity into the urine. Without sufficient salt in the body, the body will become increasingly acidic
- Salt is essential in the treatment of emotional and affective disorders. Lithium is a salt substitute that is used in the treatment of depression. To prevent suffering from depression, make sure you take some salt
- Salt is essential for preserving the serotonin and melatonin levels in the brain. When water and salt perform their natural antioxidant duties and clear the toxic waste from the body, essential amino acids, such as tryptophan and tyrosine, will not be sacrificed as chemical antioxidants. In a well-hydrated body, tryptophan is spared and gets into the brain tissue where it is used to manufacture serotonin, melatonin, and tryptamine—essential anti-depression neurotransmitters
- Salt, in my opinion, *is vital for the prevention and treatment of cancer.* Cancer cells are killed by oxygen; they are anaerobic 'organisms'. They must live in a low-oxygen environment. When the body is well hydrated and salt expands the volume of blood circulation to reach all parts of the body, the oxygen and the active and 'motivated' immune cells in the blood reach the cancerous tissue and destroy it. As I explained in my book on lupus, dehydration—shortage of water and salt—suppresses the immune system and its disease-fighting cells' activity in the body
- Salt is vital for maintaining muscle tone and strength. Lack of bladder control in those who suffer from involuntary leakage of urine could be a consequence of low salt intake. Salt is most

43

effective in stabilizing irregular heartbeats and, contrary to the misconception that it causes high blood pressure, is actually essential for the regulation of blood pressure—in conjunction with water. Naturally, the proportions are critical. A low-salt diet with high water intake will, in some people, actually cause the blood pressure to rise. *As a secondary complication, it can also cause asthma-like shortness of breath.* The logic is simple. If you drink water and do not take salt, the water will not stay in the blood circulation adequately to completely fill all the blood vessels. In some, this will cause fainting, and in others, it will cause tightening of the arteries—*and eventually constriction of bronchioles in the lungs*—to the point of registering a rise in blood pressure, complicated by breathlessness. One or two glasses of water and some salt— a little of it on the tongue—will quickly and efficiently quieten a racing and 'thumping' heart, *and in the long run,* will reduce the blood pressure and cure breathlessness

- Salt is vital for sleep regulation. It is a natural hypnotic. If you drink a full glass of water, then put a few grains of salt on your tongue, and let it stay there, you will fall into a natural, deep sleep. Don't use salt on your tongue unless you also drink water. Repeated use of salt by itself might cause nose bleeds
- Salt is a vitally needed element in the treatment of diabetics. It helps balance the sugar levels in the blood and reduces the need for insulin in those who have to inject the chemical to regulate their blood sugar levels. Water and salt reduce the extent of secondary damage associated with diabetes
- Salt is vital for the generation of hydroelectric energy in all of the cells in the body. It is used for local power generation at the sites of energy need by the cells
- Salt is vital to the communication and information processing of nerve cells the entire time that the brain cells work—from the moment of conception to death
- Salt is vital for the absorption of food particles through the

intestinal tract
- Salt is vital for clearing the lungs of mucus plugs and sticky phlegm, particularly in asthma, emphysema and cystic fibrosis sufferers
- Salt on the tongue will stop persistent dry coughs
- Salt is vital for clearing up catarrh and sinus congestion
- Salt is vital for the prevention of gout and gouty arthritis
- Salt is essential for the prevention of muscle cramps
- Salt is vital in preventing excess saliva production to the point that it flows out of the mouth during sleep. Needing to constantly mop up excess saliva indicates salt shortage
- Osteoporosis, in a major way, is the result of salt and water shortage in the body
- Salt is absolutely vital to making the structure of bones firm
- Salt is vital for maintaining self-confidence and a positive self-image—a serotonin- and melatonin-controlled 'personality output'
- Salt is vital for maintaining sexuality and libido
- Salt is vital for reducing a double chin. When the body is short of salt, it means the body really is short of water. The salivary glands sense the salt shortage and are obliged to produce more saliva to lubricate the act of chewing and swallowing and also to supply the stomach with water that it needs for breaking down foods. Circulation to the salivary glands increases and the blood vessels become 'leaky' in order to supply the glands with more water to manufacture saliva. This 'leakiness' spills to areas beyond the glands themselves, causing increased bulk under the skin of the chin, the cheeks and into the neck
- Salt is vital for preventing varicose veins and spider veins on the legs and thighs
- Sea salt contains about 80 mineral elements that the body needs. Some of these elements are needed in trace amounts. Unrefined sea salt is a better choice of salt than other types of salt on the market. For instance, ordinary table salt has been

stripped of its companion elements and contains additive elements such as aluminium silicate to keep it powdery and porous. Aluminium is a very toxic element in our nervous system. It is implicated as one of the primary causes of Alzheimer's disease

- As much as salt is good for the body in asthma, excess potassium is bad for it. Too much orange juice, too many bananas, or any 'sports drink' containing too much potassium might precipitate an asthma attack, particularly if too much of the drink or too many bananas are taken before exercising. It can cause an exercise-induced asthma attack. To prevent such attacks, some salt intake before exercise will increase the lungs' capacity for air exchange. It will also decrease excess sweating

- It is a good policy to add some salt to orange juice to balance the actions of sodium and potassium in maintaining the required volume of water inside and outside the cells. In some cultures, salt is added to melon and other fruits to accentuate their sweetness. In effect, these fruits contain mostly potassium. By adding salt to them before eating, a balance between the intake of sodium and potassium results. The same should be done to other juices

- I received a call one day from one of the readers of my book to tell me how he had unwittingly hurt his son. Knowing that orange juice was full of vitamin C, he forced his son to drink several glasses of it every day. In the meantime, the young boy developed breathing problems and had a number of asthma attacks until he reached college and moved out of the sphere of influence of his father. His asthma cleared and his breathing became normal. The father told me he had to call his son and apologize for having given him such a hard time when he was younger. The more the son had rebelled against orange juice, the more the father had insisted he should take it, convinced a large amount was good for him

- As a rough rule of thumb, you need about 3 grams of salt—a

46

half-teaspoon—for every 10 glasses of water, or a quarter teaspoon per quart of water. You should take salt throughout the day. If you exercise and sweat, you need more salt. In hot climates, you need to take even more salt. In these climates, salt makes the difference between survival and better health and heat exhaustion and death

- **Warning! You must at the same time not overdo salt.** You must observe the ratio of salt and water needs of the body. You must always make sure you drink enough water to wash the excess salt out of the body. *If your weight suddenly goes up in one day, you have taken too much salt.* Hold back on salt intake for one day and drink plenty of water to increase your urine output and get rid of your swelling
- *Those in heart failure – or kidney failure requiring dialysis – MUST consult with their doctors before increasing salt intake.*

Asthma and allergy

'One deceit needs many others, and so the whole house is built in the air and must soon come to the ground.' - **Baltasar Gracian**

The National Library of Medicine in Bethesda, Maryland, held an exhibition on asthma in 1999. The mission statement of the exhibition and the historical progress of our present understanding of asthma were presented to show that, although the disease has been around for thousands of years, its outcome has not changed. More people suffer from and die of asthma today than ever before. But the exhibition was designed to say that 'we have made progress; we now have so many medications designed to help asthmatics'. Nowhere was there any indication that the 'system' is in search of understanding the cause and finding a natural cure for asthma. The focus is on asthma management. To show that something substantial is being done, research is said to focus on the discipline of genetics to pinpoint the disease!

Asthma and allergy—conditions mainly treated with different kinds of antihistamine medications—are important indicators of dehydration in the body. Histamine is a most important neurotransmitter that primarily regulates the thirst mechanism for increased water intake. It also establishes a system for rationing the available water in the body during dehydration. Histamine is a most noble element employed in the drought management of our bodies. In dehydration, histamine production and its activity increase greatly. Increased histamine release in the lungs causes the spasm of the bronchioles. This natural spasmodic action of histamine on the bronchial tubes is part of the design of the body to conserve water that would normally evaporate during breathing. The winter steam or fog that you see when you breathe out in cold weather is water that is leaving your lungs as you breathe.

We breathe approximately 720 times an hour. Imagine how much water we lose through breathing in one hour, in one day, in one week! Could we live for long if we did not replace the water loss from our lungs? When we neglect to replace this water loss, how does the body deal with this crisis? Initially, and stage by stage, the drought management programs of the body are activated. In some, bronchial constriction—asthma—is the first reaction to dehydration. Children are more susceptible to asthma than adults. Their bodies are growing all the time and every cell in an expanding body needs 75 percent of its volume in water. At the same time, children's bronchial trees are smaller and less rigid, and can be constricted more efficiently than fully developed bronchial trees with firm cartilage support in their structure. Children's bodies also have less of a water reserve to tap into for redistribution. These are the reasons children exhibit shortness of breath—asthma—more readily than adults when they become dehydrated.

Attacks of asthma during exercise and stress are also part of the water preservation and crisis management process during dehydration. An asthma attack after eating is a classic indicator of dehydration. If we eat food and don't drink water in order to digest and 'liquefy' the food we have stuffed into the stomach, the water that is needed to complete the digestion process is borrowed from the rest of the body. This repeated scrounging of water from here and there in an already drought-stricken person predisposed to asthma will precipitate an asthma attack. Both emotional and physical stress cause more acute dehydration to an already dehydrated body. The 'free' water that is available for new functions is utilized very rapidly in the chemical reactions needed to cope with any particular form of stress.

Take action
You can naturally prevent asthma and allergy by drinking more water. When you understand the physiology of the human body and

the role of histamine in its water regulation and drought management, you realize that chronic dehydration in a vast majority of people is the primary cause of allergies and asthma. Increased water intake—*on a forced, regular basis*—should be adopted as a preventive measure as well as the treatment of choice. In those who have had attacks of asthma or allergic reactions to different pollens foods, more strict attention to daily water intake should become a pre-emptive measure. These people will also have other indicators of dehydration they need to recognize and treat accordingly before a crisis attack of asthma endangers their lives and exposes them to possible, premature death. Don't forget, the chemical pathways dealing with dehydration have no 'brain'; they rush forward like a cascade. They are actually called 'chemical cascades'. These dehydration-induced chemical cascades kill many thousands of asthmatics a year. They are easily 'turned off' by water and salt, two strong, natural antihistamines.

How much water should you drink?

If you suffer from allergies and asthma, you should begin drinking water daily on a regular basis, and take salt regularly too. You should stop taking caffeine and alcohol in your drinks, at least until your condition has become normal. Always remember that some fluids may not be a suitable replacement for simple water, particularly for children. People with normal heart and kidney function should begin drinking two glasses of water a half-hour before each meal, and one glass of water two and a half hours after the meal. *Drink water any time you feel thirst, even in the middle of a meal.* Remember, children need water for cell growth. Naturally, smaller children need less water than grown-ups. A rough rule of thumb of how much water a person needs is half one's body weight in ounces of water every day. A 60-pound child then will need about 30 oz of water [approx 4 x 8 oz glasses]. Some children might need 3/4 of their body weight in ounces of water. They will also need to take some extra salt.

As we age, we lose our thirst sensation and do not recognize our bodies are thirsty. Chronic dehydration in the elderly can cause heart and kidney damage. Those with heart problems and kidney disease, and who are under treatment, should increase their water intake slowly and, if possible, under the supervision of their physician. Urine production should increase with additional water intake. If, within two full days, there is no indication of more urine being produced, a physician should be consulted. The colour of urine in a dehydrated person (who is not taking B vitamins that can colour the urine) is dark yellow to orange. In a better hydrated person, the urine is lighter in colour.

Children and adults who get asthma attacks with exercise and strenuous effort should always remember to drink water before they begin exercising and to stop drinking caffeine-containing sodas. *They should also take some salt before exercise*—salt will increase stamina during exercise. They should reduce their orange juice intake (if more than two glasses). Because of its high potassium content, orange juice in large quantities can predispose a sufferer to an asthma attack. The water needs of the body cannot be fully replaced by juices or other potassium-containing beverages. The same applies to milk. It is safer to add a little salt to the orange juice to balance the sodium/potassium intake when one wants to drink orange juice.

Using water and salt for allergies

For extensive allergic reactions, one should immediately drink at least three or four glasses of water and take a little salt to prevent circulation problems that can occur when circulation to the skin increases to the point of producing skin eruptions, blotchiness, and even oedema or swelling. In this situation, water and salt will act as very strong antihistamines and increase urine production so that the toxic material causing the eruptions can be flushed out.

At the same time, exposing the skin to water from the outside, such as by showering or bathing, will help alleviate the itchiness and other symptoms. The best way to deal with this situation is to stand under a shower and change the water from hot to cold every minute. The water should be as hot and as cold as you can bear. By doing this, you will exhaust the chemical reserves of the local nerves and ultimately abort the reactive response of the nerve endings on the skin. Normally, five to ten minutes of hot and cold showers, ending with a cold shower, will take away itchiness completely.

Let me tell you about a case I treated in this way. A young man, 24 years old, had become allergic to something in his food and had developed a rash that covered him from the top of his head to almost his toes. He had an uncontrollable itch and desire to scratch, which had caused skin damage. He responded to this hot and cold method of treatment within minutes and his skin irritation ceased to bother him.

Using water on the outside of the body has medicinal values in many conditions. For example, if you are starting a cold, this treatment works well and is used in Scandinavian countries all the time. This is the logic behind saunas so popular in that region. People sit in the sauna to heat their bodies and then jump into an ice-cold pool.

My recommendation is that anyone taking a hot shower should finish up with a cold shower. In this way, the body will become much more adept at dealing with the stresses of environmental temperature fluctuations. For years, I started my day with a cold shower, and I did not have one day of sickness, a cold or flu. I mention this way of dealing with allergies in order to show that, even in extreme cases, water can be effective very quickly.

Dyspepsia/heartburn

'We concentrate on consistency without much concern of what it is we are being consistent about, or whether we are consistently right or wrong. As a consequence, we have been learning a great deal about how to follow an incorrect course with the maximum of precision.' – **W Deutscher, University of Manchester Institute of Science and technology course hand-out**

The dyspeptic pain is the most important signal for the human body. It denotes dehydration. It is a thirst signal. It can occur in the very young as well as in older people. Chronic and persistently increasing dehydration is the root cause of almost all currently encountered major diseases of the human body.

Of the dyspeptic pains, that of gastritis, duodenitis and heartburn should be treated with an increase in water intake alone. When there is associated ulceration(s), attention to daily diet to enhance the rate of repair of the ulcer site becomes necessary.

It is generally understood that 12 percent of those with dyspepsia develop ulceration in their duodenum after six years, 30 percent after 10 years and 40 percent after 27 years. It is the dyspeptic pain that is of significance, although the condition develops importance once the ulceration is viewed through the endoscopic examination. It seems that medical practice is becoming more and more a visually oriented discipline rather than the perceptive and thought-based art it was at one time.

It is the pain associated with these differently classified conditions that forces the person to consult a medical practitioner. It is this pain that is now getting much attention even though many different jargons are attached to the local conditions seen through the endoscope. The common factor is the dyspeptic pain. The local tissue change is the descriptive explanation for the changes brought about by the basic common factor, namely the initiating dehydration.

How am I able to make such claims? I have treated with only water well over 3,000 persons with dyspeptic pain, who had other distinguishing characteristics to classify them according to those jargons. They all responded to an increase in water intake and their clinical problems associated with the pain disappeared. The report of my new way of treating dyspeptic pain with water was published as the editorial article in the *Journal of Clinical Gastroenterology* in June 1983.

At a certain threshold of dehydration, when the body urgently calls for water, nothing else can substitute. No medication other than water is effective. One of the many patients I treated with water proves this fact. He was a young man in his middle twenties. He had suffered from peptic ulcer disease for a number of years before the crisis time, when I met him. He had the usual diagnostic procedures performed on him and received the label of 'duodenal ulcer'. He had been given antacids and brand name cimetidine medications.

Cimetidine is a very strong medication that blocks the action of histamine on its '2nd' type receiver points, generally known as 'receptors' in the body; in this case, known as histamine 2 or H_2 receptor. It just happens that some cells in the stomach that produce the acid are sensitive to this medication. However, many other cells in the body that do not produce acid are also sensitive to this blocking action of the medication. That is why this medication has many other side-effects, (including impotence in the young) and has proven extremely dangerous in the chronically dehydrated older age group.

The first time I set eyes on the young man was at eleven one evening in the summer of 1980. He was in such pain, he was almost semiconscious. He was folded in the foetal position on the floor of his room. He was groaning steadily, unaware of his environment and the worried people around him. When I talked to him, he did not respond and was not communicating with those around him. I had to shake him to get a response. I asked him what the matter was. He groaned, "My ulcer is killing me." I asked him how long he had experienced the pain. He said it had started at one in the afternoon immediately after his lunch. The pain increased in intensity during the afternoon. I asked him what had he done to get relief and if he had taken any medication. He replied that he had taken three tablets of cimetidine and one whole bottle of antacid during this time. He indicated that he got absolutely no relief even with this amount of medication in the ten hours since his pain first started.

When so much medication could not relieve the pain of peptic ulcer disease, one automatically becomes suspicious of 'acute abdomen', something that might possibly need surgical exploration. Maybe his ulcer had perforated! I had seen and assisted in the operation of patients with perforated peptic ulcers. Those persons were devastated—very much like the young man before me. The test is very simple; such patients develop a very rigid abdominal wall, almost like a wooden board. I felt for the rigidity of the wall of the abdomen in this young man. Fortunately, he had not perforated. His abdominal wall was soft, but tender from the pain. He was lucky he had not perforated, although if he had continued like this, the acid would have punched a hole through his ulcer.

The choice of medications in such circumstances is very limited. Three cimetidine tablets of 300 milligrams each and one full bottle of antacid had not relieved the pain. Often, such cases end up on the operating table of a knife-happy surgeon. Because of my extensive experience with the pain-relieving properties of water in dyspeptic pains, I gave this man two full glasses of water—one pint. At first he was reluctant to drink the water. I told him he had taken the usual medications without any result. He should now try 'my medication' for this disease. He had no choice. He was in severe pain and did not know what to do about it. I sat in a corner and observed him for a few minutes.

I had to leave the room but when I returned fifteen minutes later his pain had become less severe and his groans stopped. I gave him another full glass of water—half a pint. In a few minutes, his pain disappeared completely and he started taking notice of the people around him. He sat up and began to move toward the wall of the room. With his back to the wall, he started to conduct conversations with his visitors who were now more surprised than he was at the sudden transformation three glasses of water had brought about! For ten hours this man had suffered from pain and taken the most potent and advanced medicines for the treatment of peptic ulcer disease without any relief. Now, three glasses of water had produced total relief in about twenty minutes.

After a certain threshold, local painkillers will not be effective. The antacid and H2 blocking agent cimetidine did not produce even a reduction in the pain felt by the young man. It was water alone that registered the right message with the brain to abort its call for water, since there was now an unmistakable signal of its adequate presence in the body. The same mode of pain registration is operative in the other regions that signal dehydration in any particular individual. People with rheumatoid joint pain should be aware of this particular phenomenon of pain registration at the brain when there is severe dehydration.

I had another occasion to test whether the abdominal pain registration for dehydration was time-dependent or water volume-dependent. This time, a man was carried by two other persons into the clinic where I was working at the time. The patient could not walk. He too was an old peptic ulcer patient in extremely severe upper abdominal or dyspeptic pain. After examination to see that he had not perforated, I gave the patient one full glass of water every hour. He did not achieve total relief in twenty minutes, or even one hour and twenty minutes. He recovered after he had taken three glasses of water. On the average, it takes less severe cases about eight minutes to achieve total pain relief.

It has been shown experimentally that when we drink one glassful of water, it immediately passes into the intestine and is absorbed. However, within one half-hour, almost the same amount of water is secreted into the stomach through its glandular layer in the mucosa. It swells from underneath and gets into the stomach, ready to be used for food breakdown. The act of digestion of solid foods depends on the presence of copious amounts of water. The acid is poured on the food, enzymes are activated, and the food is broken down into a homogenized fluid state that can pass into the intestine for the next phase of digestion.

The mucus covers the glands' layer of the mucosa, which is the innermost layer of the structure of the stomach. Mucus consists of 98 percent water and 2 percent the physical 'scaffolding' that traps water. In this 'water layer' called mucus, a natural buffer state is established. The cells below secrete sodium bicarbonate that is trapped in the water layer. As the acid from the stomach tries to go through this protective layer, the bicarbonate neutralizes it.

The outcome of this action is a greater production of salt (sodium from the bicarbonate and chlorine from the acid). Too much salt alters the water-holding properties of the 'scaffolding' material of mucus. Too much acid neutralization and salt deposits in this mucus layer would make it less homogeneous and sticky and would allow the acid to get to the mucosal layer, causing pain.

The natural design in the re-secretion of water through the mucus layer seems to be the process of 'back-washing' the mucus layer and getting rid of the salt deposits. This is a most efficient design for rehydrating the mucus layer from the bottom when new mucus is also secreted. This refreshed, thickened and sticky mucus barrier is the natural, protective shield against the acid in the stomach. Naturally, the efficiency of this shield depends on a regular intake of water, particularly before the intake of different, solid foods that would stimulate the production of acid from the glands in the stomach wall. Thus, water provides the only natural protection against the acid in the stomach, from base upward. Antacids are designed to attach to the acid in the stomach itself—an inefficient protection.

We should begin to realize that in the same way we have a 'hunger pain' signal, we also have a 'thirst pain' signal in the body. It is unfortunate they call it 'dyspepsia' and treat it with all sorts of medications until there is local duodenal or stomach tissue damage from the metabolic complications of dehydration. The use of antacids for the relief of this pain is generally the accepted form of treatment. These substances are non-prescription slow poisons that one can buy even in the supermarkets.

Significant research conducted in Sweden has shown that the outcome is the same in those who do not have an actual ulcer and yet have the classical dyspeptic pain, whether or not they use a placebo, an antacid or even the agent that blocks the action of histamine. In other words, neither antacid nor the stronger medication are all that effective. It is at this stage of body physiology, now generating signals of dehydration, that one should be prudent and refrain from the use of any form of medication.

Water is most probably the only effective substance to give relief. After all, water and only water is what the body wants, needs and is calling for. If we search accurately for other signs, there would be more indicators of dehydration. Do not imagine that dyspeptic pain is the indicator of an isolated and localized phenomenon. In any case, dyspeptic pain is a signal of dehydration—a thirst signal—of the body, even if there is an associated ulcer. If water is taken and it relieves your pain, with adequate food intake, the ulcer is bound to repair itself in due course.

Other Digestive Complaints

'Never does nature say one thing and wisdom another.' - **Juvenal**

Helicobacter pylori

It is now said that ulcers are the result of infections. My researched opinion is that the variety of curved bacteria blamed for causing ulcerations are commensals – bacteria that naturally dwell in the intestines. They may take unfair advantage of the immune system suppression that is the direct outcome of dehydration. You see, the normal intestinal bacteria cohabitate with us and produce much of the vitamins needed by the body. They contribute to our well-being when we are strong. In dehydration, particularly at the site of the valve between the stomach and the duodenum, many histamine-producing nerves exist. This particular curved bacterium, *helicobacter pylori,* benefits from the growth hormone effects of histamine at the same time that these nerves are restrictively monitoring the rate of flow of the strongly acid content of the stomach into the intestine. In any case, not all ulcer sites show the presence of 'helicobacters', and contrariwise, people may have helicobacter in their intestines and not suffer from ulcers.

Antacids

Antacids that contain aluminium are dangerous. They should not be freely used for a condition that will respond to an increase in water intake. Excessive aluminium in circulation has been strongly implicated as a precipitating factor on top of other considerations in Alzheimer-type disease. It is imperative to understand this relationship between taking aluminium-containing antacids for a long period of life and possible, accumulative, toxic side-effects of brain damage in Alzheimer's disease. No amount of genetic study will undo the toxic side-effect of a metal used in medications to deal with a simple signal of thirst under the wrong paradigm. Most antacids contain between 150-600 milligrams of aluminium in every spoonful of the liquid, or in each tablet that is chewed.

The island of Guam has much aluminium ore in its soil (normally the case for some regions in the Western Pacific—Guam island, Kii peninsula in Japan, Western New Guinea and others). The drinking water of the island was heavily contaminated with aluminium. During the time this contamination was not recognized and remained in the drinking water, a disease similar to Alzheimer dementia was prevalent on the island. Even the younger people on the island seemed to suffer from the disease. A number of years later this problem was recognized and the water purified. It has been noticed that the younger people seem not to be afflicted any more. It is now taken for granted that it was the aluminium in the drinking water that caused an Alzheimer-type dementia on the island of Guam.

Anti-histamine medications

Histamine-blocking agents are also not suitable for long-term use. They have many side-effects. These include dizziness and confusion states in the elderly. Enlarged breasts appear in men after a few weeks of taking this medication. Low sperm count in some male patients and loss of libido have also been noted. Nursing mothers or pregnant women should not use this type of medication to treat the thirst signals of the body—both the child's and the mother's. The brain capillaries respond to dehydration by dilating if histamine stimulates them. These antihistamines will block the capillary-dilating action of histamine when the brain has to tabulate more information than normal—the pressure of stress. The brain will get less blood supply when antihistamines are used for dyspeptic pain treatment.

Colitis pain

Colitis pain, felt in the lower left part of the abdomen, should initially be viewed as another thirst signal for the human body. It is often associated with constipation, itself caused by persistent dehydration.

One of the main functions of the large intestine is to remove water from the excrements to avoid losing too much of it in defecation after food digestion. When there is dehydration, the residue is naturally devoid of the normal amount of water necessary for easier passage. Also, by slowing down the flow, even the final drops of water will be drawn away from the solid residue in the large gut. Thus, constipation will become a complication of dehydration in the body. With added food intake, more solid waste will be packed into the intestine and increase the burden for passage of its hardened waste content. This process will cause pain. Colitis pain should initially be considered as a thirst signal of the body. With adequate water intake, the left lower abdominal pain that is associated with constipation will disappear. Eating an apple, a pear, or an orange in the evenings will help reduce constipation in the next day.

False appendicitis pain

A severe pain can sometime appear in the lower right abdominal region. It can mimic an inflammation of the appendix and present some similarity to the pain of early appendicitis. Other distinguishing characteristics are not seen; there is no rise in body temperature; there is no guarding in the abdominal wall and no feeling of nausea. One or two glasses of water will relieve this lower right abdominal pain. One glass of water can serve as a diagnostic tool in this particular condition.

Hiatus hernia

You often come across the classical dyspeptic pain that the doctor has diagnosed as hiatus hernia. Hiatus hernia means displacement of the upper part of the stomach through the gap in the diaphragm into the chest cavity. This would be an unnatural place for the stomach to be in. With a part of the stomach in the chest, food digestion becomes painful.

Normally, the content of the upper part of the stomach is sealed off and cannot pass upward into the oesophagus when food is being digested. The normal direction of intestinal contractions is downward, from the mouth to the rectum. Furthermore, there are two valves that prevent the regurgitation of food upward. One is located in the wall of the tract between the oesophagus and the stomach. This valve only relaxes when food is going into the stomach. The other trap valve is located outside of the tract in the diaphragm, where the oesophagus passes through it to join the stomach. This valve is synchronized to relax every time the food that is being swallowed in the oesophagus has to pass through it. At other times it is tight and does not permit the content of the stomach to pass upward. This is the normal state of affairs for the two 'valves' which prevent the passage of food from reversing direction and passing upward.

The intestinal tract, from the mouth to the rectum, is a long tube. Different parts of it have special physical and functional attributes to make the process of food digestion and evacuation of waste a well integrated and smooth operation. There are many local hormones that make this operation possible. Local hormones are chemical messengers that time the next stage of the process to 'kick in'. They cause the necessary enzymes to be secreted to promote further breakdown and subsequent absorption of the active materials in food.

Early in the process of digestion, acid is secreted in the stomach to activate the enzymes and help in the breakdown of solid proteins such as meat and hard-to-digest foods. Normally, liquefied but highly acidic content of the stomach is pumped into the first part of the intestine. There is a valve between the stomach and the intestine known as the 'pyloric valve'. Its operation is regulated by the message system from either sides of the 'tract'. It is one thing for the stomach to wish to empty its contents into the intestine, it is another for the intestine to be ready to receive this highly corrosive and acidic, gastric content.

The pancreas is a gland that secretes insulin to regulate blood sugar and also pours essential digestive enzymes into the intestine. *It has at the same time the physiological responsibility of rendering the intestinal environment alkaline before the acid from the stomach can reach the intestine.* This most important function of the pancreas involves manufacturing and secreting a watery bicarbonate solution, which neutralizes the acid as it enters the intestine. To manufacture the bicarbonate solution, the pancreas needs much water from the circulation. In dehydration, this process is not very efficient. For this reason, the pyloric valve will not receive the clear signals to open and allow the stomach acid to pour into the intestine. This is the first step in the production of dyspeptic pain, the initial thirst indicator of the human body.

When we drink water, depending on the volume of water that enters the stomach, a hormone/neurotransmitter called 'motilin' is secreted. The more water we drink, the more motilin is produced by the intestinal tract and can be measured in blood circulation. The effect of motilin on the intestinal tract, as its name implies, is to produce rhythmic contractions of the intestines - peristalsis - from its upper to lower end. Part of this action involves the timely opening and closing of the valves that are in the way of flow of intestinal content.

Thus, when there is enough water in the body for all the digestive processes that depend on the availability of water, the pancreas will produce its watery bicarbonate solution to prepare the upper part of the intestinal tract to receive the acidic content of the stomach. Under such ideal circumstances, the pyloric valve is also allowed to open for the evacuation of the content of the stomach. Motilin has a major 'transmission' role in coordinating this action. *Motilin is a satiety hormone. It is secreted when water extends the stomach wall.*

The problem begins when there is not enough water in the body for these digestive events to take place in their coordinated manner. In no way will the system allow the corrosive contents of the stomach to reach the intestine if the mechanism to neutralize is not effective. The damage would be irreparable. The walls of the intestines do not possess the same protective layer against acid available to the stomach. The first thing that happens is the reversal of the strength of contraction in the valves on either side of the stomach. The pyloric valve will constrict more and more.

The ring valve between the oesophagus and stomach and the external 'valve' of the diaphragm will become more relaxed. Initially, some of the acid may flow into the oesophagus when the person is lying down and produce a type of pain named 'heartburn'. In some, the laxity of the valve in the diaphragm may be such that a portion of the stomach may pass through it into the chest and achieve the title of hiatus hernia. When the valves reverse their mode of operation for the normal flow of stomach content, in effect they are preparing for another eventual and unavoidable outcome – the evacuation of the stomach content through the mouth. If the stomach content cannot go into the intestine and it cannot indefinitely remain in the stomach, there is only one other way out - through the mouth. For this action to take place, the intestinal tract is capable of reversing the direction of its contractions. The reversal of the contractions is termed 'anti-peristalsis'.

In my opinion, because of the repeated corrosive effect of the regurgitating acid on the unprotected oesophageal tissue, there is a strong relationship between heartburn of early life and eventual cancer of the lower end of the oesophagus.

Dyspeptic pain, no matter what other pathological label is attached to it, should be treated with regular intakes of water. The current treatment practice and the use of antacids and histamine-blocking agents are not to the benefit of a chronically dehydrated person whose body has resorted to crying for water.

A.B. is herself engaged in alternative medicine. She is very strongly into chelation therapy. She has compiled information and written a book on chelation. However, she had herself suffered for many years from excruciating pains from her hiatal hernia. Her husband, himself a most delightful author, tells me that A.B. could hardly sit through a meal and not suffer from such severe pains as to be able to complete her food and enjoy sitting down for a chat. At times, they would have to leave the restaurant because the pain would not allow her even a short respite to finish her meal.

A.B tells me she hardly drank any water. After Harold had by chance come across my book and read it, they soon understood A.B's problem. She began drinking water. As she increased her water intake she noticed her pain was less severe. In a matter of days it disappeared completely, never to come back. The husband and wife now enjoy going out to eat. My wife and I ate with them a few times. It appears her hiatal hernia and its pain are now ancient history.

Bulimia

I am sure you are very sympathetic to people who have been given the label of 'bulimic'. These people eat and then throw up whatever they have eaten. The most famous bulimic was probably the late Princess Diana. Bulimia sufferers are constantly hungry and are also depressed and antisocial, as seems to have been the case with Princess Diana throughout her private and married life.

There is a belief among pundits who profess to understand bulimia that the whole problem is caused by an undercurrent of psychological issues within the thought processes of bulimics. Since more women suffer from the problem than men, it is assumed that the act of eating and then throwing up is a measure to remain thin. I disagree.

Uncontrollable and repeated vomiting of the stomach contents, which has been given the medical labels of 'heartburn' or 'bulimia', could be one of the ways the body prevents irreparable damage when it is severely dehydrated. When it is said that bulimics feel hungry all the time, there is confusion. As far as I am concerned, they are confusing their sensation of thirst with hunger. When they should be drinking water, they eat. Naturally, the body rejects the food because it does not possess enough water to digest and assimilate the food. This is the reason why bulimics grow so thin. The same dehydration can also be responsible for some of the emotional and psychological changes in these people.

I met Amir in the prison where I started to research the impact of water on the treatment of peptic ulcer disease. For more than ten years, on and off, he had been suffering from heartburn. During the flare-up phase of the problem, he would routinely vomit in his sleep - so forcefully that part of his stomach contents would jet out of his nose. Often he could not clear out of his bed in time to avoid making a mess. You can imagine he had difficulty sleeping during these times. Because none of the regular medications could stop such vomiting, he had taken it for granted that his problem was incurable.

I asked him to drink a full glass of water half an hour before his food and increase his daily water intake. As simply as you read these lines, his heartburn disappeared and never came back while he was in the prison with me.

Let me share with you the human side of Amir's story. It is interesting that in his immediate family, his daughter, his wife, and his brother had similar problems - heartburn that culminated in vomiting when the disease flared up. At this time in the life of the family, when there was a lot of fear that Amir might not get out of prison soon, none of them was in a good state of health. They were stressed beyond words. They would travel for miles every week to see Amir. They would wait outside the prison walls for hours in the heat of the summer and cold of the winter, to have a ten- to fifteen-minute visitation.

On one of these occasions, he shared with them the fact that increased water intake had cured him of his 'disease'. He was jubilant that now his family could do the same. One by one they got rid of their devastating heartburn and the social complications they had experienced for many years. Luck was with Amir. He was released unexpectedly. Before he left, he came to me and thanked me for what I had done for him. He told me, *"It was worth coming to prison to get cured of my disease!"*

Summary
An inaccurate assessment of digestive problems as a thirst signal will later in life cause the human body many irreversible problems. Of course, a stomach tumour could cause a similar pain. However, that pain will not disappear with water, it will continue to recur. In case there are repeated pains even when water intake has been regulated for a number of days, it would be prudent to consult a physician for assessment of the condition. If the pain is from gastritis and duodenitis, or even peptic ulcerations, the regular intake of water is a must in the daily routine and dietary adjustments for the treatment of these conditions.

High blood pressure

'Physicians think they are doing something for you by labelling what you have a disease.' – **Immanuel Kant**

High blood pressure (essential hypertension) is the result of an adaptive process to a gross body water deficiency.

The vessels of the body have been designed to cope with fluctuation of their blood volume and tissue requirements by opening and closing different vessels. When the body's total fluid volume is decreased, the main vessels also have to decrease their aperture (close their lumina), otherwise there would not be enough fluid to fill all the space allocated to blood volume in the design of that particular body. Failing a capacity adjustment to the 'water volume' by the blood vessels, gases would separate from the blood and fill the space, causing 'gas locks'. This property of lumen regulation for fluid circulation is a most advanced design within the principle of hydraulics and after which the blood circulation of the body is modelled.

Shunting of blood circulation is a normal routine. When we eat, most of the circulation is directed into the intestinal tract by closing some capillary circulation elsewhere. When we eat, more capillaries are opened in the gastrointestinal tract and fewer are open in the major muscle systems. Only areas where activity places a more urgent demand on the circulatory systems will be kept fully open for the passage of blood. In other words, it is the blood-holding capacity of the capillary bed that determines the direction and rate of flow to any site at a given time.

This process is naturally designed to cope with any priority work without the burden of maintaining an excess fluid volume in the body. When the act of digestion has taken place and less blood is needed in the gastrointestinal region, circulation to other areas will open more easily. In a most indirect way, this is why we feel less active immediately after a meal and ready for action after some time has passed. In short, there is a mechanism for establishment of priority for circulating blood to any given area - some capillaries open and some others close. The order is predetermined according to a scale of importance of function. The brain, lungs, liver, kidneys and glands take priority over muscles, bones and skin in blood distribution *unless* a different priority is programmed into the system. This will happen if a continued demand on any part of the body influences the extent of blood circulation to the area, such as muscle development through regular exercise.

Water shortage: potentials for hypertension

When we do not drink enough water to serve all the needs of the body, some cells become dehydrated and lose some of their water to the circulation. Capillary beds in some areas will have to close so that some of the slack in capacity is adjusted for. *In water shortage and body drought, 66 per cent is taken from the water volume normally held inside the cells; 26 per cent is taken from the volume held outside the cells; and 8 per cent is taken from blood volume.* There is no alternative for the blood vessels other than closing their lumina to cope with the loss in blood volume. The process begins by closing some capillaries in less active areas. The deficient quantity must come either from outside or be taken from another part of the body.

It is the extent of capillary bed activity throughout the body that will ultimately determine the volume of circulating blood. The more the muscles are exercised, the more their capillaries will open and hold a greater volume of blood within the circulation reserves. *This is the reason why exercise is a very important component for physiological adjustments in those suffering from hypertension.* This is one aspect to the physiology of hypertension. The capillary bed must remain open and full and offer no resistance to blood circulation. When the capillary bed is closed and offers resistance, only an increased force behind the circulating blood will ensure the passage of some fluids through the system.

Another reason why the capillary bed may become selectively closed is shortage of water in the body. Basically, water we drink will ultimately have to get into the cells – water regulates the volume of a cell from inside. Salt regulates the amount of water that is held outside the cells – the ocean around the cell. There is a very delicate balancing process in the design of the body in the way it maintains its composition of blood at the expense of fluctuating the water content in some cells of the body.

When there is a shortage of water, some cells will go without a portion of their normal needs and others will get a predetermined, rationed amount to maintain function (as explained, the mechanism involves water filtration through the cell membrane). However, blood will normally retain the consistency of its composition. It must do so in order to keep the normal composition of elements reaching the vital centres.

This is where the solutes paradigm is inadequate and goes wrong. It bases all assessments and evaluations of body functions on the solids content of blood. It does not recognise the comparative dehydration of some other parts of the body. All blood tests can appear normal and yet the small capillaries of the heart and the brain may be closed and cause some of the cells of these organs a gradual damage from increasing dehydration over a long period of time. When you read the section on cholesterol formation, this statement becomes more obvious.

When we lose thirst sensation (or do not recognise other signals of dehydration) and drink less water than the daily requirement, the shutting down of some vascular beds is the only natural alternative to keep the rest of the blood vessels full. The question is, how long can we go on like this? The answer is, long enough to ultimately become very ill and die. Unless we get wise to the paradigm shift, and professionally and generally begin to recognise the problems associated with water metabolism disturbance in the human body and its variety of thirst signals, chronic dehydration will continue to take its toll both on our bodies and our society.

Essential hypertension should primarily be treated with an increase in daily water intake. The present way of treating hypertension is wrong to the point of *scientific absurdity*. The body is trying to retain its water volume, and we say to the design of nature in us: 'No, you do not understand - you must take diuretics and get rid of water!' It so happens that, if we do not drink sufficient water, the only other way the body has to secure water is through the mechanism of keeping sodium in the body. Only when sodium is retained will water remain in the extra-cellular fluid compartment. From this compartment, through the mechanism of 'shower-head' production, water will be forced into some of the cells with priority status. *Thus, keeping sodium in the body is a last resort way of retaining some water for its 'shower-head' filtered use.*

There is a sensitivity of design attached to sodium retention in the body. To assume this to be the cause of hypertension is inaccurate and stems from insufficient knowledge of the water regulatory mechanisms in the human body. When diuretics are given to get rid of the sodium, the body becomes more dehydrated. The dry mouth level of dehydration is reached and water is taken to compensate. Diuretics maintain the body at an expanding level of deficit water management. They do not cure hypertension; they make the body more determined for salt and water absorption, but never enough to correct the problem. That is why, after a while, diuretics are not enough and supplemental medications will be forced on the patient. Another problem in assessment of hypertension is its means of measurement. *Anxiety associated with having hypertension will automatically affect the person at examination time!* Readings of the instruments may not reflect the true, natural and normal blood pressure. An inexperienced or hasty medical practitioner, more in fear of litigation than mindful of accuracy of judgement, might assume the patient to have hypertension, whereas the person might only have an instant of 'clinic anxiety', thus causing a higher reading of the instrument.

One other very important but less-known problem with the mechanism of reading blood pressure is the process of inflating the cuff well above the systolic reading, and then letting the air out until the pulse is heard. Every large (and possibly small) artery has a companion nerve to monitor the flow of blood through the vessel. With the loss of pressure beyond the cuff that is now inflated to very high levels, the process of 'pressure' opening of the obstruction in the arteries will be triggered. By the time the pressure in the cuff is lowered to read the pulsation level, the recording of an artificially induced higher blood pressure will have become unavoidable. Unfortunately, the measurement of hypertension is so arbitrary (and based on the diastolic level) that in this litigious society a minor error in assessment may label a person hypertensive. This is when the fun and games begin.

Water by itself is the best natural diuretic. If people who have hypertension and produce adequate urine increase their daily water intake, they will not need to take diuretics. If prolonged 'hypertension-producing dehydration' has also caused heart failure complications, water intake should be increased gradually. In this way, one makes sure that fluid collection in the body is not excessive or unmanageable. The mechanism of sodium retention in these people is in overdrive. When water intake is increased gradually and more urine is being produced, the oedema fluid (swelling) that is full of toxic substances will be flushed out, and the heart will regain its strength.

Higher blood cholesterol

'The whole aim of practical politics is to keep the populace alarmed, and hence clamorous to be led to safety, by menacing it with an endless series of hobgoblins, all of them imaginary.'
– H L Mencken

Higher blood cholesterol is a sign that the cells of the body have developed a defence mechanism against the osmotic force of the blood that keeps drawing water out through the cell membranes; or *the concentrated blood cannot release sufficient water to go through the cell membrane* and maintain normal cell functions. Cholesterol is a natural 'clay' that, when poured in the gaps of the cell membrane, will make the cell wall impervious to the passage of water (see Figure 14 overleaf).

Its excessive manufacture and deposition in the cell membrane is part of the natural design for the protection of living cells against dehydration. In living cells that possess a nucleus, cholesterol is the agent that regulates permeability of the cell membrane to water. In living cells that do not possess a nucleus, the composition of fatty acids employed in the manufacture of the cell membrane gives it the power to survive dehydration and drought. Cholesterol production in the cell membrane is part of the cell survival system. It is a necessary substance. *Its excess denotes dehydration.*

Normally it is water that instantly, repeatedly and transiently forms into adhesive sheets and binds the hydrocarbon bricks together. In a dehydrated membrane, this property of water is lost. At the same time that water is binding the solid structure of the membrane, it also diffuses through the gaps into the cell.

I have presented this researched concept at an international gathering of cancer specialists. These same scientific statements are published and have been discussed by other researchers. How does this phenomenon affect us in our everyday life? The answer is simple. Imagine that you are sitting at a table and food is brought to you. If you do not drink water before you eat the food, the process of food digestion will take its toll on the cells of the body. Water will have to be poured on the food in the stomach for proteins to break and separate into the basic composition of their amino acids. In the intestine, more water will be required to process the food ingredients and then send them to the liver.

In the liver, the specialised cells will further process the intestine-digested materials and then pass *the resupplied and composition-adjusted blood* to the right side of the heart. In the liver, more water is used to process the food ingredients. The blood from the right side of the heart, which has also received some 'fat' components from the lymphatic system that empties into the right side of the heart, will now be pumped into the lungs for oxygenation and exchange of the dissolved gases in the blood. In the lungs, aeration of the blood further dehydrates it by the process of evaporation of water - the 'winter steam'.

Now this highly concentrated blood from the lungs is passed to the left side of the heart and pumped into the arterial circulation. The first cells that will face this highly osmotically concentrated blood are the cells lining the larger blood vessels and capillaries of the heart and the brain. Where the arteries bend, the osmotically damaged cells will also face the pressure of the oncoming blood. Here, the cells will either need to protect themselves or become irreversibly damaged. Do not forget that the integrity of their cell membrane is proportionately dependent on the presence of water available to them and not that which is being osmotically pulled out.

There comes a moment when the brain begins to recognise the further imposed severe shortage of water in the body, and then, in the middle of eating food, the person will feel compelled to drink. It is already too late because the damage is registered by the cells lining the blood vessels. However, when this dehydration registers itself by production of the dyspeptic pain, we most stupidly give the person antacid! Not water - antacids! Not water - histamine-blocking agents! Unfortunately, this is the problem with all treatment procedures under the solutes paradigm.

All treatment procedures are oriented towards the relief of symptoms. They are not geared to the elimination of the root cause of the problem. This is why 'diseases' are not cured, they are only 'treated' during the lifetime of the person.

The root cause of degenerative diseases is not known because a wrong paradigm is being pursued. If we begin to appreciate that for the process of food digestion *water is the most essential ingredient,* most of the battle is won. If we give the necessary water to the body before we eat food, all the battle against cholesterol formation in the blood vessels will be won.

After a longer period of regulating daily water intake, so that the cells become fully hydrated, gradually the cholesterol defence system against the free passage of water through the cell wall will be less required; its production will decrease. The hormone-sensitive, fat-burning enzymes of the body have been shown to become active after one hour's walk. They remain active for 12 hours. It also seems that with the lowering of blood cholesterol and walking to induce the 'fat burners' activity, deposited cholesterol will also be broken and passage of blood through the already blocked arteries will become possible.

Walking twice a day every 12 hours will maintain the activity of the hormone sensitive fat burning enzyme (hormone sensitive lipase) during day and night and help clear away the excess lipid deposits in the arteries.

Everyone who has raised blood cholesterol levels is worried. It is common knowledge that many diseases are associated with raised cholesterol levels in blood circulation. Different blood cholesterol levels have, in the past, been considered normal - all the time decreasing the accepted threshold until around 200 (milligrams per 100 cubic centimetres of blood) is now considered normal. Even this figure is an arbitrary assessment.

I personally believe the normal range to be around 100 to 150. My own levels started around 89 and never went above 130. Why? Because for years and years, my day started with two to three glasses of water. In any case, a March 28, 1991 *New England Journal of Medicine* report, followed by an editorial about an 88-year-old man who eats 25 eggs daily and has normal blood cholesterol levels, reveals one fact. The cholesterol we eat seems to have little to do with the high level of cholesterol in some people's blood.

Let us get one thing clear: *excess cholesterol formation is the result of dehydration.* It is the dehydration that causes many different diseases and not the level of cholesterol in the circulating blood. It is therefore more prudent to attend to our daily water intake rather than to what foods we eat. With proper enzyme activity, any food can be digested, including its cholesterol content. Anyone can reduce their cholesterol levels without too much anxiety about their food intake. All you have to do is drink more water before your meals. If you take regular daily walks, cholesterol levels will further reduce during the following months.

If increased water intake lowers cholesterol levels, only to rise again, make sure your body is not getting short of salt. The importance of this has already been explained. You should realise that cholesterol is the basic building block for most hormones in the human body. Naturally, a basic drive for increased hormone production will also raise the rate of cholesterol production.

Basically, it is assumed that heart disease begins with the deposit of cholesterol plaques in the arteries of the heart. At the final stages, the two may exist at the same time. However, in my opinion, it begins when the constriction producing chemicals from the lungs spill over into the circulation that goes to the heart.

As with asthma, in dehydration, part of the process of water preservation is the associated secretion of substances that constrict the bronchioles. At a certain threshold that does not at the time manifest itself in an asthma attack, the same chemicals, if they spill into the blood circulation that goes through to the lung, will also constrict the walls of the heart arteries once they reach them. This situation will lead to heart pains, known as anginal pains.

These same chemicals can also set the stage for the deposit of cholesterol in the walls of the arteries. The common factor to all of the various conditions labelled as different diseases of the heart and the lungs is an established dehydration.

Water is a readily available natural medicine for some prevalent and very serious medical conditions that are known to kill many thousands of people every year. Is it heart disease or dehydration that is killing people? In my professional and scientific view, it is *dehydration* that is the biggest killer, more than any other condition you could imagine. The different physiological aspects and 'chemical idiosyncrasies' of each individual's body reaction to the same pattern of dehydration have received different professional labels and have been treated differently - *and ineffectively.*

Dehydration is the common factor. It is the difference in the 'chemical blueprint' in the design of each person's body that initially demonstrates signs of chronic dehydration by producing different outward indicators.

Later in the process, other indicators of the same dehydration problem become apparent. The reason for this difference in the initial pattern may be the selective process of 'shower-head' emergency hydration of some cell types in the body. If you read the testimonies at the end of this book, you will see certain individuals had multiple problems that got better by the regulation of daily water intake.

You are now privy to information on where the mistake lies in the creation of monstrous problems within the healthcare systems in scientifically advanced countries. They seem to allow for the arrogant treatment of a simple dehydration of the human body by chemical mallets until real diseases are born.

Obesity
How dehydration causes excess weight
(You overeat when you are thirsty!)

The sensations of thirst and hunger are generated simultaneously to indicate the brain's needs for energy supply. We do not recognize the sensation of thirst and interpret both indicators as the urge to eat. We eat food even when the body should receive water, the infinitely cleaner source of energy.

Storage of energy in the energy pools in the brain, and in the absence of adequate generation of hydroelectricity, seems to rely heavily on the availability of sugar. The brain has constantly to collect sugar from the blood to replenish its ATP and GTP stockpiles.

In our society, we have developed a sweet tooth for immediate satisfaction of the brain. Many cultures, such as the Chinese, have avoided this cultural pitfall. In the West, however, we consume a lot of sugary foods. In such situations when the body receives a good supply of 'sweetness', the liver begins initially to store the extra sugar in form of starch, and subsequently in form of fat. Glycogen is made of a very long chain of glucose molecules that are connected together in the form of a 'polymer'. It is stored in the liver and muscle tissue. Glycogen is the readily usable starch that can very quickly be converted – one or two glucose molecules at a time – into ATP when the ATP reserves of the cells in the body are beginning to get depleted.

Since only 20 per cent of the circulation reaches the brain, only 20 per cent of the sugar in circulation is used up; the remaining 80 per cent is stored in the liver and fat cells. Beyond what the liver stores as glycogen, excess sugar is converted into fat and released into the blood circulation to be stored by the fat cells. Fat cells also collect sugar and convert it to fat independently of the liver. This is why I call food taken for brain energy 'dirty fuel'. In normal circumstances, food should be balanced for the repair of wear and tear and the manufacturing needs of the body, and not as the primary and only source of brain energy — the brain exercises priority for its needed supplies over the rest of the organs in the body. Water should be available to manufacture 'local' hydroelectricity for the constantly active brain cells.

Water breaks down fat

Fat is a high-energy product that is stored in different tissues to be used when the energy supply from outside the body becomes erratic or diminished. Fat is stored in specially designed fat cells that pick up the excess sugar in circulation and convert it to fatty acids, which are lumped together to form triglycerides – chunks of fat. To reuse this stored fat, it has to be broken back into individual fatty acids once again and released as free fatty acids in circulation to be picked up by the tissues that are short of energy. Breakdown of fat depends on the presence of water. One unit of water has to be sacrificed to separate one unit of fatty acid from its connection to the 'chain'. The process is called hydrolysis of fat. Hydrolysis of fat is under the control of an enzyme called lipase. This is why we need to drink water regularly and often to supply its free form for the breakdown of fat. Water will also indirectly stimulate the lipase that breaks up fat.

To understand the fat-breakdown process in relationship to eating, you need to understand the following physiological events:

- Lipase gets activated when the level of sugar available to fat cells falls lower than is normally present in circulation.

- Peaking the blood sugar by the intake of sweet snacks or starchy foods, which immediately get converted to sugar and cause insulin release, will inhibit lipase activity.

- Lipase activity is also brought about by the release of many hormones and neurotransmitters. This variety of lipase is known as hormone-sensitive lipase. Adrenaline and noradrenaline (norepinephrine) are by far the most potent of the lipase activators. Growth hormone, other adrenal gland hormones and thyroid hormone are other potent activators of lipase.

- In the absence or very short supply of carbohydrates, and when the stored glycogen is getting used up, the body preferentially metabolizes fat from its stores for energy formation.

- Normally, 40 to 50 per cent of the calories in a good diet are from fat. In any case, much of the carbohydrate eaten is converted into fatty acids and metabolized gradually throughout the day, unless the system is loaded with successive carbohydrate intake. Often, this is the result of confusion between feeling thirsty and hungry, when you eat instead of quenching your thirst with water.

- The energy formed from one molecule of sugar is much less than the energy formed from one molecule of fat. One gram-molecule of sugar forms 38 units of ATP from 66 per cent of energy in the sugar, and the other 34 per cent is converted to heat; one molecule of fat forms 146 units. Thus, fat burning is more energy-efficient than burning carbohydrates. Think about it: The body knows how to store energy. What we want to do is learn how to tap into that energy without letting it accumulate excessively to the point of distorting the shape of the body. Water seems to be the ideal 'solution' for this problem.

- The liver is fully capable of de-saturating fatty acids for ready use in the architectural structure of membranes. The triglyceride content of the liver consists mainly of its unsaturated variety, whereas the rest of the fat stores of the body are formed from the saturated fatty acids. This information brings into question the validity of the conventional views on essential fatty acids, even though in the past I have also subscribed to those views. Here you see the true value of an open mind in scientific research. I no longer worry about the kind of fat I eat. I enjoy my generous helpings of butter with the knowledge that my liver will take care of the rest.

- Fat is a most important element for human survival. In the water environment of the interior of the body, fat plays an indispensable and vital insulating role as fatty acids, cholesterol and phospholipids. Both starch and proteins are water-soluble and will not be able to protect the architecture of the cells from getting out of shape and distorted.

- Eighty per cent of cholesterol formed in the liver is eventually converted into bile salts, secreted into the biliary tract, and passed on into the intestine. The other 20 percent is converted into phospholipids and passed into the blood circulation.

- Cholesterol, apart from its use in the cell membrane of the brain and nerve tissues, is further converted into most of the sex hormones, secondary neurotransmitters (such as the array of prostaglandins, prostacyclins and thromboxane) and vitamin D. Cholesterol further acts as an insulating bandage over abrasions and tears in the inner membrane of the arterial walls that get damaged because of the rush of 'concentrated' pulsating blood, which becomes acidic and possibly corrosive when the body becomes dehydrated. What you see as cholesterol plaques in the arterial system of blood circulation has never been seen in the veins of the body. This simple explanation reveals that the reasons offered for pushing cholesterol-lowering medication on people in our commerce-driven society are based more on fraud than science.

- All the cells of the body can use fatty acids interchangeably with glucose for energy. Thus, if the body has no problem burning fat, why do we insist on giving it more carbohydrate than fat? Even brain cells, after a few weeks, can learn to derive up to 50 to 75 per cent of their energy from fat instead of sugar.

- This is the reason the body stores 150 times more energy in the form of fat than glycogen (starch).

- For each 9.3 calories of excess energy, 1 gram of fat will be deposited in the fat stores.

- About one-third of energy in normal people goes into muscle activity. In physically active people, as much as three-quarters of the energy consumed could be used for maintaining muscle activity. Thus, physical activity that engages the main muscle mass in the body is the best way to tap into the energy reserves of the body stored in its fat deposits.

- The total amount of stored starch in the entire body that will get used up in dieting or starvation is around a few hundred grams – good for only about half a day. Fat and proteins follow suit, fat more quickly than proteins. But loss of proteins could be detrimental, particularly as some of the more vital essential amino acids get attacked and become depleted through their use as antioxidants.

- The onset of some serious diseases begins with the loss and depletion of the essential amino acids.

84

When muscles are inactive, their energy stores are more easily attacked, and even their protein reserves are ultimately broken down for conversion into sugar. However, if muscles are used, they begin to metabolize some of their stored fat as a choice source of energy to do work and maintain or increase their bulk. To do this, they begin to activate the fat-breaking enzyme, hormone-sensitive lipase. Repeated blood tests in a company of Swedish soldiers on a three-week march showed that this enzyme's activity is seen after one hour's walk; it remains in circulation and retains its fat-breaking activity for 12 hours. The activity of the enzyme becomes cumulative with increased walking. The soldiers showed very strong activity of their hormone-sensitive lipase throughout their march.

Why is this information significant? As you know, the bulk of our bodies' muscle content is located in the legs and hips, the anatomical parts used in locomotion. Also significant is the fact that burning fat for locomotion is economical: One gram of fat provides more than twice as much energy for muscle activity as the equivalent weight in sugar or protein. Remember, one gram of fat generates 9 calories of energy whereas 1 gram of sugar or of protein provides 4 calories. Burning fat is the most efficient way for the muscles to use the body's energy stores. Thus, making and retaining fat is the most efficient way to establish an energy reserve for the body to be used at times of scarcity, such as in winter. This information alone indicates that we are wrong in reducing the fat in our diets; instead, we should eat more healthy oils and fat and less carbohydrate.

Water and fat storage

There is an inverse relationship between water consumption and fat accumulation in the body. The less water you drink, the more you will be forced to eat. The more you eat, unless you are physically active, the more you store fat. Here are the reasons:

- Water is the primary source of energy for all physiological functions of the body.

- Water turns 'micro-electric turbines' — the cation pumps — and generates electricity for neurotransmission and nerve impulses in the entire body.

- Every food item that has to be broken down and metabolized will need the chemical influence of water – hydrolysis – before its energy can be utilized by the cells of the body. In effect, water transfers its hidden energy to the substances it breaks down, as previously mentioned, increasing their energy content by about one order of magnitude.

- In cell membranes, water is used for its stickiness – like the ice that sticks to your fingers – and acts as the adhesive that holds membrane structures together. In dehydration, the stickiness of cholesterol has to hold and insulate the cell membrane – hence we see a gradual rise in cholesterol levels from increased food intake when the body is dehydrated.

- The constant communication of nine trillion brain cells is energy-dependent and must be powered by either hydroelectric energy or energy from the metabolism of food. Excess energy from hydroelectricity is stored in the form of ATP, and the extra water leaves the body in the form of urine. It does not form a 'lake' in the body. Excess energy from food taken to maintain brain activity is stored in the form of fat – only 20 per cent of 'solid' energy from food reaches the brain, while the rest is stored as fat, unless used in physical activity.

- The early sensation of thirst and sensation of hunger – stemming from low brain energy levels – are similar. They get reflected in heartburn/hunger pang sensations. We never recognized heartburn as an indicator of thirst until I treated 3,000 people suffering from the heartburn of peptic ulcer disease with only water. I later proved this sensation to mean thirst for water. We traditionally treated this sensation, before it became severe, as though it were only a hunger pain – hence overeating when the body is actually thirsty. This confusion is the background to getting fat – we eat more food, even before full digestion of earlier meals, hence indigestion, gas formation and bloating. Taking a glass of water before eating and allowing time for the satiety mechanism to kick in corrects this mistake. A glass of water will work more efficiently than any antacid or gas-reducing medication.

- Taking a glass of water before eating also stimulates secretion of adrenaline and noradrenalin by the sympathetic system for at least two hours. This direct action of water on the sympathetic nervous system forcefully activates hormone-sensitive lipase to break down fat for use as energy to enhance the physical activity of the body. This is the reason water overrides the sensation of hunger in a short period of time.

- The human body recycles and constantly circulates around 40,000 glasses of water in every 24 hours (from information published by Loma Linda University in California). If each glass of water is 250 cc or 8 ounces, then the circulation is hauling about 10,000 litres or 2,500 gallons of water every 24 hours. This physiological function is intensely energy-consuming – hence the release of energy from the fat stores of the body through the sympathetic nervous system activation of lipase when we drink water.

- Thus, water has two strong direct effects in preventing the body from becoming obese. Firstly, by providing 'clean' energy for brain function, it avoids the storage of fat from excess food intake. Secondly, by constantly activating the fat-burning enzymes, water tips the balance in favour of breaking up the fat reserves when the body is going through the process of recycling its fat stores. This is the reason people who choose the WaterCure lose weight without any effort.

- One advantage of adequate hydration for reducing fat stores is the fact that you don't need to count calories. Your taste buds and the satiety mechanism of your body will do the work for you.

- After you drink a glass of water, for up to two hours it will stimulate the secretion of one of the gut's dominant hormones, motilin. Motilin acts exactly like serotonin. Serotonin, in turn, is the chief of all neurotransmitters in the brain; it regulates all the brain's physiological responses to outside stimulation. Serotonin is what depressed people do not have enough of. They take medications to protect its presence in their bodies. Normal people have enough serotonin in their brains and nerve systems. When water stimulates the release of motilin, it is in fact causing the brain to know that water is on board and thirst is quenched. Motilin is a satiety hormone.

- Motilin does yet another thing: It activates motility in the intestines and promotes passage of their contents downstream. It acts as a laxative. Thus, two glasses of water first thing in the morning will be a more effective intestinal stimulant and a lubricating laxative than anything you might imagine - and it is all natural and what the body wanted all the time. Your body will not need to squeeze the contents of its guts for their last drop of water, making what should be routine bowel movements painful events.

- The satiety action of motilin will overcome any sensation you might interpret as hunger. This is the reason why people who want to diet and lose weight need to drink water before any food and give it time to override their perception of hunger. What's happening is simple: Water provides hydroelectric energy for the brain, and the low energy sensation of the brain that is commonly interpreted as 'hunger' is cancelled. At the same time lipase, activated by the sympathetic nervous system, will shunt the metabolic direction of the body into fat breakdown and its conversion into energy – the same ATP that you would make from sugar. 'The quick fix with sugar' for the panic-stricken brain will not be needed if you drink your next glass or two of water.

- The regular intake of water will keep the physiology of your body in its fat-breaking mode until you take your next sugary or starchy food. These encourage insulin-induced fat storage and 'hypoglycemic panics' (cravings) that force you to eat more of the same. To overcome this problem, it is more prudent to eat protein snacks that might even be high in their fat content. Do not be frightened of some fat in your diet. It is not the fat content of your diet that causes heart disease. It is chronic unintentional dehydration – and its associated mineral deficiencies – that is the primary cause of heart problems.

- Remember, when your daily diet does not include adequate water, you do not properly absorb the minerals in your food. This is when the body becomes acidic, and acidic blood eats into the delicate arterial membranes. You need water and minerals to get rid of the acidic waste products of metabolism in the urine you pass out – the light colour of urine is a good indicator of an alkaline body. Dark yellow or orange urine means an acidic body, the primary indicator of the onset of heart disease.

How to lose weight naturally

Water is a natural medication for people who tend to put on weight. To lose already gained weight, water is more effective than anything in the arsenal of the drug or diet industry. When you give water a chance to fulfil its primary role in bodily energy formation, your natural desires for food will shift from starch to protein and fat, and your cravings for sugary stuff will be few and far between.

The next step would be to add muscle activity to enhance the action of water on the fat-breaking enzyme lipase. If you wish to lose weight as a crash course, two walking sessions – one in the morning and one in the evening – will activate lipase around the clock, even while you sleep. Not only will you begin to lose fat from your body, but you will also clear the cholesterol 'bandage' from the acid-damaged walls in your arteries that can now get repaired – a welcome fringe benefit.

Fat stores in the body also collect some of the toxic chemicals that foods are sprayed or prepared with. When fat is released for energy, you need the extra water to wash out these released chemicals. You also have to pay attention to your minerals and salt intake to keep all the pumps active for hydroelectric energy formation.

I suppose you would now like to hear some reports on the effectiveness of proper hydration as a means of losing weight. There are some success stories at the end of this book. As you'll see, when you correct the dehydration of the body, not only do you lose weight, but you also get rid of many other disease complications of dehydration. Most of the people who lost 20, 30 or 40 pounds did not start the programme of re-hydration of their bodies to lose weight; they were focusing on their other health problems such as asthma, hypertension, back pain and more. They were not dieting to lose weight. Their weight loss was the natural outcome of hydrating their bodies.

And what of the people who were out to lose weight? Their loss was so impressive that it surprised everyone around them. They lost their excess pounds without hassle or too much effort. The kind of loss that was achieved with increased water intake is the kind for which some people undergo drastic, mutilating surgery. The long-term outcome of such operations is not yet known. One thing is for sure, though: If there are problems ahead, unfortunately the surgery cannot be reversed.

So you now understand the role of water in weight regulation. What you might need in addition is strong willpower to overcome the urge to feast on sweet stuff. All you need to do is to stand in front of the mirror and tell yourself you want to be slimmer than you are. Create an image of a smaller you in your mind and revisit this image over and over again until your mind is made up. Your brain is a very sophisticated computer. It will begin to programme its chemical demands and controls on the basis of the newly installed programme [patterning] in its subconscious mind. After you have made sure your brain knows a slimmer you is what you want, you will automatically avoid all the goodies you ate in the past. Make sure you give your body ample water, some vital minerals and salt for their essential energy-making activities. It is my professional understanding that most overweight people are subconsciously compelled to overeat to obtain their sodium and other mineral needs. Unfortunately, they do not realize that they also need water to absorb these minerals.

There are two important points to remember:

1.   You need to prevent thirst to lose weight. When you wait to get thirsty to drink water, you get confused and think you are actually hungry, even if you ate only two or three hours ago. When you are fully hydrated, the constructive effect of food will last, and it will be a long time before you're hungry again. You should quench your thirst with water; manufactured and taste-enhanced beverages sweetened to make them marketable defeat the purpose and turn off the fat-burning enzymes.

2. When you reduce your food intake and increase your water intake to lose weight, supplement your diet with vitamins and minerals. You must make sure you do not become deficient in those minerals which you would normally get from your food. Also, be sure to use unrefined salt from the ocean or old salt mines in the mountains [Himalayan] – not the regular table salt that is stripped of its companion minerals. Salt and mineral cravings force you to overeat.

Lastly - satiety mechanisms

Fat tissue is also an endocrine gland. It produces many hormones. One of these is called lepitin. Lepitin is supposed to let the brain know when the fat reserves are fully replenished. Obviously, in fat people, the mechanism is ineffective. I do believe proper hydration corrects this discrepancy between lepitin levels in blood circulation and their proper assessment by the brain cells.

Another satiety mechanism is connected to the stretch sensors in the stomach. This is when the brain realizes enough is enough. The more we eat and force the stomach to stretch, the more the brain becomes insensitive to the message system from the stretch sensors in the stomach. The brain gets used to the over-stretching of the stomach tissue – this is the case with all fat people.

The most effective and least understood food intake control mechanism is attached to the taste buds on the tongue. This control system can only work when food is held in the mouth as long as possible while chewing it. The taste buds register with the brain the volume and type of food that has been processed and passed through. The slow rate of chewing – until the food is totally minced into very small particles, and even liquified by its mixing with saliva, gives the brain time to calculate the energy value of what has passed into the stomach – the satiety mechanism takes over and possible overeating will stop. Try it!

Phillip Day: The elimination cycle, one of three eight-hour digestive cycles your body moves through every twenty-four hours, commences around 4am and ends at noon. Try avoiding heavy digestion during this period (the classic 'breakfast'), enabling the body to concentrate its resources on shedding weight (elimination) as part of its normal metabolic processes. Drinking water in the morning upon rising sets your body up for the day and promotes fat metabolism. Vegetable shakes are also fine during this period, requiring minimal energy expenditure for digestion, and bringing with them an impressive payload of minerals, enzymes and amino acids.

Try commencing your eating cycle (appropriation) from noon until 8pm, leaving the final 8pm – 4am period for 'assimilation', when the body conducts its metabolic housekeeping during your horizontal sleeping hours.

Depression

'What you don't know can hurt you.'
Samuel Epstein MD

Perceptive markers of dehydration

Dr Batmanghelidj: When the body becomes dehydrated, the brain can still get water delivered by 'raindrops' through the filter system in its cell membranes but this is not enough to energize it as fully as when the body is hydrated. This discrepancy in the rate of water supply to the brain produces a certain number of sensory outcomes that I consider thirst perceptions. They are as follows:

Thirst perceptions
- Feeling tired
- Feeling flushed
- Feeling irritable
- Feeling anxious
- Feeling dejected
- Feeling depressed
- Feeling inadequate
- Feeling a 'heavy head'
- Cravings
- Agoraphobia

This list should help you recognize the earlier stages of depression before it becomes deeply established. Bear in mind that ultimately tiredness could be an early marker of depression. When you are too tired to get out of bed first thing in the morning, you are, in fact, so dehydrated that your brain is refusing to get engaged in your daily routine. Water up and don't let the problem turn into full-blown depression.

What is depression?

If it is the hot season and you are too preoccupied to water your grass, it will die of 'brown grass disease'. First the grass wilts, then patches of it begin to go yellow and then brown. If these symptoms of dehydrated grass do not register in your mind the need to get out the water hose and thoroughly soak the yard, all the grass in your charge will die. And if, God forbid, the importance of water as a medication against the browning of grass and foliage is not held in the safekeeping of your brain, you might wonder what specialist could come and save you from having to re-grass your lawn. And, since specialists are by nature hard to come by and expensive, you would have no choice but to listen to their pearls of wisdom, particularly if the occurrence of brown grass disease is thought to be a genetic problem of the grass in your garden.

You would have no choice but to have the whole area of brown grass dug up and replanted with a different strain of grass. Since your new grass has to be watered to grow, you come away with the idea that your specialist knows what he's talking about, and totally in the dark that even your old grass needed to be watered regularly to stay green.

In its early stages, depression is like the brown grass disease of the brain cells. It is a direct outcome of not drinking water on a regular basis and, worse, of drinking caffeinated beverages in place of water. Caffeine is a drying agent and dehydrates the body. Nine trillion brain cells need water all the time. The brain is 85 per cent water and needs every drop of it to perform its most complicated functions. Depression is much like the wilting stage of brown grass, but sadly you cannot dig up the brain cells and plant new gene-improved models in their place, at least not yet. You will have to make do with what you have – so water it.

Depression is only a label given to the physiological state of a dehydrated brain that is not able to perform all its sophisticated functions. Depending on what area of the brain is more affected by dehydration, different subsets of labels have been generated for the same basic problem. And because jargon-peddling is the way of 'knowledgeable professionals', the simple shortage of water, and the material resources it would bring with it for the needs of the brain, has been responsible for the creation of psychiatry as a field among the medical disciplines. The difference between psychology and psychiatry is in the way the patient is treated. In the one discipline they talk you out of your concerns, and in the other they medicate you into conformity.

Since you have been initiated into the field of psychiatry by the advertising programmes of the drug industry, you likely want to know all about the relationship of water to serotonin and its reuptake inhibitors and so on, before you can begin to value water as an effective natural medication against depression.

The amino acid link to depression

There are 20 amino acids. From these, the body manufactures different proteins for construction of both body tissues and the active messenger agents that regulate the body's functions. The body has the ability to manufacture 10 of these amino acids but the other 10 cannot be manufactured and must be imported. The 10 amino acids the body can make are alanine, glycine, proline, serine, cysteine, aspartic acid, glutamic acid, asparagines, glutamine, and tyrosine. However, at least two of these amino acids – cysteine and tyrosine – are derivatives of other essential amino acids that the body cannot manufacture but must consume. Cysteine is manufactured from methionine, and tyrosine is manufactured from phenylalanine.

The body can manufacture some histidine, but not enough of it during childhood and old age. For this reason, histidine should also be considered an essential amino acid. The essential amino acids – listed in the order of their importance for brain function – are histidine, tryptophan, phenylalanine, methionine, lysine, threonine, valine, arginine, leucine, and isoleucine.

Histidine gets converted to the neurotransmitter histamine and is responsible for the water regulation and resource management of the body. It operates your thirst sensations and regulates the water-rationing programmes of the body. It is with us from minute one of life when the ovum is fertilized by the sperm, but has not yet divided into the two cells. Histamine has to 'wet-nurse' the ovum for it to be able to expand in volume and then divide, and divide, until the baby is born - histamine is there all the time. In childhood, when the body is growing, histamine acts as a strong growth factor, much like growth hormone. The difference is that histamine becomes more and more active as we grow older, while growth hormone activity diminishes very rapidly from the third decade of life.

The tremendous need for the actions of histamine in childhood and old age makes its precursor amino acid, histidine, essential. Many neurological disorders, such as multiple sclerosis, seem to be produced because of histidine metabolism imbalance. Many emotional problems are associated with excess activity of histamine during its water-regulation.

The more the body becomes dehydrated, the more histamine activity takes over the physiological functions that were the responsibility of water. If there is not enough water to energize the mineral pumps, or cation pumps, and regulate the balance between sodium (which has to stay outside the cells) and potassium (which must be forced back in), histamine stimulates the release of energy to jump-start the protein pumps and bring about osmotic balance in the environment of the cells – most vitally in the brain.

Histamine acts as a natural energy manager in the absence of water and shortage of hydroelectric energy. Brain function is not efficient without histamine when the body is short of water. Nor is it efficient for long if it has to rely only on histamine as a substitute for the functions of water. In essence, this state of inefficient brain physiology, caused by the missing action of water, is what we call depression. Histamine is in charge of the ionic balance inside the cells. It forces potassium ions that leak out of the cell wall back into the cell. It releases energy for the pumps that handle the process. The trigger mechanism that gets histamine going is a rise in the level of potassium in the environment around the cells, particularly the brain cells. In my opinion, the action of histamine in the body is what preserves life until water becomes available and can perform its natural functions. The use of antihistamine medications, when water itself is a better natural anti-histamine, is tantamount to a criminal act. The tricyclic antidepressant medications, and in fact even the more modern antidepressants, function as very strong antihistamines.

The essential amino acid tryptophan gets converted into at least four neurotransmitters and hormones: serotonin, tryptamine, indolamine, and melatonin. Two enzymes, one unique to serotonin-producing cells and the other distributed more generally in the brain, act on tryptophan in this conversion process. Nature has selected tryptophan as the most important amino acid for the brain's control of all the sensations and functions of the body.

Serotonin is the kingpin chemical, needed for many events that silently regulate the body physiology. This is why a shortage of the serotonin that should normally be available is one of the hallmarks of depression. It's also why the pharmaceutical industry has produced a number of chemicals that slow down the rate of serotonin's destruction in the nerve terminals after it is secreted to perform one of its many functions:

- Serotonin alters the threshold of pain sensation and produces analgesia.
- Serotonin controls production and release of the growth hormone.
- Serotonin controls the level of blood sugar.
- Serotonin controls the blood pressure levels of the body - it has a tendency to lower blood pressure.
- Serotonin and tryptophan control appetite. You remember I talked about motilin, which is considered a kind of gut serotonin. It is the hormone that causes the satiety sensation.
- Serotonin and tryptophan regulate the body's salt intake, whereas histamine controls the intake of potassium and its insertion into the cells.
- Serotonin has a direct effect on calcium movement into the cells and its involvement in neurotransmission.
- Serotonin release inhibits histamine's release and its action.
- Serotonin production by the brain is reduced when the blood levels of three amino acids – valine, leucine, and isoleucine – rise above normal, such as in starvation, dehydration, lack of exercise, and other conditions that affect protein metabolism of the body.
- Serotonin strengthens the contractile properties of certain muscles.
- The serotonin-stimulated nerve system (serotonergic system) is the medium through which analgesics such as morphine and hallucinogenic drugs like LSD register their effects. It is this kind of stimulation of the serotonergic system that becomes addictive when people get hooked on a drug, be it caffeine or cocaine.

The brain cells that convert tryptophan to serotonin have the ability to make this conversion at the same rate as it arrives. These cells do not store tryptophan itself, but store serotonin in vesicles and even pass these vesicles on the nerves' transport system down the track to the nerve endings, to be used when the nerve is stimulated. Thus, low serotonin levels in the nerve system – seen in depression – are only caused if tryptophan cannot be delivered to the nerve cells.

You now understand the physiological upheaval that occurs as a result of tryptophan shortage in the brain tissue. After 20-plus years of research into the relationship of water to pain regulation of the body, I have reached a broad understanding of how to avoid serotonin depletion in the brain and prevent depression.

Water: nature's antidepressant medication

Directly or indirectly, water maintains an efficient and effective rate of tryptophan flow into the brain tissue for its immediate conversion into serotonin. Here's how:

- Normally, when the body gets dehydrated and cannot produce adequate urine to get rid of its toxic waste and the acid build-up in its cells, certain amino acids are sacrificed to neutralize this acid and make the body more alkaline. The term usually used is antioxidant. Tryptophan, tyrosine, cysteine, methionine and more are all sacrificed in an attempt to keep the acid-alkali balance of the body chemistry within the normal range.

- Drinking enough water to create colourless urine — resulting in the washing of excess acid out of the body – would automatically conserve these essential amino acids, enabling them to perform their normal roles in the body. Thus adequate urine production, which should occur with water intake – not through the use of diuretics, caffeinated beverages, or alcoholic drinks – is a major safeguard against depression.

- All elements that need to get into the brain and reach its cells have to be carried on special transporter systems. These transporter systems are specific to various elements. Tryptophan shares its transporter system with five other amino acids: valine, leucine, isoleucine, phenylalanin and tyrosine. The rate at which tryptophan can cross the blood-brain barrier (BBB) depends on the level of these other amino acids in circulation.

- In starvation, dehydration and lack of exercise, blood levels of valine, leucine, and isoleucine increase. This reduces the available transport system for the passage of tryptophan across the BBB, thus causing a gradual depletion of the available tryptophan in the brain. If dehydration and lack of exercise become established trends in the lifestyle of any individual, the serotonin levels in the brain of that person will decrease.

- Valine, leucine, and isoleucine are energy-laden amino acids that can be used by the brain or muscle tissues for their energy needs – not to manufacture a product but rather to perform a function. Exercise enables muscle tissue to mop up these amino acids from the circulation and make an intermediate product that the liver will then complete the process and make sugar for the brain to use. As a result of the muscles' collection of these amino acids from the circulating blood, increased space on transporter system (which exists only in the capillaries that feed the brain) is made available for the amino acid tryptophan to catch a ride and reach the brain side of the circulation.

- In the same way, the rate of tyrosine transfer to the brain side of the circulation will increase and cause a build-up of the dopamine levels that complement serotonin activity in the brain for increasing motivation and purpose. Thus, adequate exercise is an effective way to replenish brain serotonin levels and ward off depression.

Another role of adequate hydration in boosting the serotonin levels of the brain is too complex to explain in this book. Briefly, tryptophan is extremely heat-excitable. Water serves the purpose by producing high heat of activation at the cell membranes. This is most effectively done at the blood-brain barrier.

This local heat excites tryptophan. It dislodges itself from the transporter protein in the blood, and attaches itself to another transporter system in the wall of the better-hydrated brain capillaries. The new transporter system in the capillary wall will more efficiently and effectively deliver it to the brain. In the brain, it gets converted to serotonin, melatonin, tryptamine, and indolamine – the chemicals that regulate entire body physiology, including your mood and outlook on life.

With its simple local heat generation, water causes a speedier shift of tryptophan into the brain. Water also has many other indirect effects that help tryptophan reach into the brain cells. Thus, water is a natural medication against depression.

To prevent disease, you must prevent dehydration from getting established in the interior of your body's cells. To reverse a disease process, you need additional insight into the metabolic complications associated with prolonged water shortage in the body. Naturally, there are other treatment pointers that need to be followed.

*   *   *   *   *

Phillip Day: Imagine the number of patients consigned to mental institutions each year with 'illnesses' of dehydration, diet and lifestyle not addressed under the current psychiatric paradigm. For that matter, consider the care homes and hospices. Patrick Holford (www.mentalhealthproject.com) has done valuable work summarising the studies examining the mental health/nutrition connection. Regarding depression, Professor Malcolm McLeod of the University of North Carolina documents that 25 – 42 percent of chronic depressives are 'atypical' and have suppressed levels of chromium.[13] The chromium element may or may not be a secondary factor in how the body executes drought management. No studies exist. If in doubt, drink water according to Dr B's recommendations, ensuring your water and salt balance is maintained over the long-term.

---

[13] www.chromiumconnection.com

Rheumatoid arthritis pain

'The worst sin toward our fellow creatures is not to hate them, but to be indifferent to them: that's the essence of inhumanity.'
- George Bernard Shaw

Dr Batmanghelidj: In the United States, about 50 million people suffer from some form of arthritis, 30 million people suffer from low back pain, millions suffer from arthritic neck pains, and 200,000 children are affected by the juvenile form of arthritis. In Britain, an estimated 20 million people suffer with joint symptoms, of whom four million are disabled because of arthritis. In addition to this, in any year, a further 20 million will have to endure back pain, with effects which range from slight inconvenience to complete incapacity.

Once any of these conditions is established in an individual, it becomes a sentence for suffering during the rest of the individual's life *unless* the simplicity of the problem's root-cause is fully understood. Initially, rheumatoid arthritic joints and their pain are to be viewed as indicators of water deficiency in the affected joint cartilage surfaces. Arthritis pain is another of the regional thirst signals of the body. In some arthritis pains, salt shortage may be a contributing factor.

The cartilage surfaces of bones in a joint contain much water. The lubricating property of this 'held water' is utilised in the cartilage, allowing the two opposing surfaces to glide freely over one another during joint movement.

Whereas bone cells are immersed in calcium deposits, cartilage cells are immersed in a matrix containing much water. As the cartilage surfaces glide over one another, some exposed cells die and peel away. New cells take their place from the growing ends that are attached to the bone surfaces on the two sides. In a well hydrated cartilage, the rate of friction damage is minimal. In a dehydrated cartilage, the rate of abrasive damage is increased. The ratio between the rate of regeneration of cartilage cells to their 'abrasive peel' is the index of joint efficiency.

Actively growing blood cells in the bone marrow take priority over the cartilage for the available water that goes through the bone structure. In the process of dilating the blood vessels to bring more circulation to the area, it is possible that the branch that goes through a tight hole in the bone cannot expand adequately enough to cope; the cells that depend on these vessels for an increased water and nutrient supply are under a physically imposed rationing control. Under such circumstances, and unless there is blood dilution to carry more water, the serum requirements of the cartilage will have to be satisfied from the blood vessels that feed the capsule of the joint. The nerve-regulated shunting mechanisms (to all the joints) also produce signals of pain.

Initially, this pain indicates that the joint is not fully prepared to endure pressure until it is fully hydrated. This type of pain has to be treated with a regular increase in water intake to produce some dilution of blood that is circulating to the area, until the cartilage is fully hydrated and repaired from its base attachment to the bone – the normal bone route of serum diffusion to the cartilage.

It is my assumption that the swelling and pain in the capsule of the joint is an indication there is dilation and oedema from the vessels that furnish circulation to the capsule of the joint. Joint surfaces have nerve endings that regulate all functions. When they place a demand for more blood circulation to the area to pick up water from the serum, the compensatory vascular expansion in the capsule is supposed to make up for the inefficiency of circulation from the bone route of supply.

Because dehydration in the joint surfaces will eventually cause severe damage – to the point of making the bone surfaces bare and exposed until osteoarthritis becomes established – the tissue damage will trigger a mechanism for remodelling of the joint. There are hormone-secreting cells in the capsule of the joint. When there is damage (also from dehydration), injured tissue has to be repaired. These local remodelling hormones take over and restructure the joint surfaces. It seems that they cater to the lines of force and pressure the joints have to endure.

Unfortunately, the repair process seems to produce a deviation of the joints. To avoid such disfigurement, one should take the initial pain very seriously and give strict attention to daily intake of water. This pain should be recognised as a sign of local dehydration. If it does not disappear after a few days of water intake and repeated gentle bending of the joints to bring more circulation to the area, one should then consult a professional practitioner of medicine.

You have nothing to lose and everything to gain by recognising the pain and the non-infectious inflammation of a rheumatoid joint as a thirst signal in your body. You are probably showing other signals of water shortage in your body, but this particular site is indicating predisposition to a more severe local damage.

If we understand the body to have difficulty in recognising its thirst state, it is possible that this lower state of alertness is also inheritable by a child. It is possible that dehydration in a rapidly growing child might also indicate its presence by the pain felt in the joints, as well as in heartburn. The mode of signal production that would denote thirst might naturally be the same in the young as in older people. It is therefore recommended that juvenile arthritis should also be treated with an increase in daily water intake.

As you can see, Dr Laurence Malone, whose letter is published at the end of this book, is an experienced medical doctor and educator. His observations on the effect of water on rheumatoid joint pains in himself show that our other colleagues in the medical profession should begin to notice the medicinal values of water in disease prevention.

Lower back pain

It should be appreciated that the spinal joints – intervertebral joints and their disc structures – are dependent on different hydraulic properties of water stored in the disc core, as well as in the end plate cartilage covering the flat surfaces of the spinal vertebrae. In spinal vertebral joints, water is not only a lubricant for the contact surfaces, it is held in the disc core within the intervertebral space and supports the compression weight of the upper part of the body. *Fully 75 per cent of the weight of the upper part of the body is supported by the water volume that is stored in the disc core; 25 per cent is supported by the fibrous materials around the disc.* In all joints, water acts as a lubricating agent and bears the force produced by the weight or tension produced by muscle action on the joint.

In most of these joints, the establishment of an intermittent vacuum promotes a silent water circulation into the joint, only for it to be squeezed out by pressure borne as a result of joint activity. To prevent back pain, one needs to drink sufficient water and do a series of special exercises to create an intermittent vacuum to draw water into the disc space. These exercises will also reduce the spasm in the back muscles that, in the vast majority of people, is the main cause of lower back pain. One also needs to adopt correct postures.

The subject of back pain and its relationship to water is so important that 1 have dealt with it in a special book, *How to Deal With Back Pain and Rheumatoid Joint Pain,* and a complementary film, *How To Deal With Back Pain.* If you get back pain and, in particular, sciatic pain, you will benefit by reading this book and seeing the film. In a majority of cases, sciatic pain can be totally relieved within half an hour when the special movements that produce an intermittent vacuum in the disc spaces – as shown in the book and film – are performed.

Neck pain

Bad posture, keeping the head bent for long periods when writing, working at a low bench, the 'freeze position' while at the computer for many hours, a bad pillow or too many pillows can be contributory factors in the production of neck pain, or even the displacement of the intervertebral discs in the neck. Neck movement is essential for the establishment of adequate fluid circulation within the disc spaces in the neck. The weight of the head forces water out of the discs over a period of time. To bring back the same water, the force of vacuum has to be created within the same disc space. This can only be done if the head and neck are moved adequately backward. A simple process in less severe cases of neck pain from disc displacement would be slowly and *repeatedly* bending the head and neck backward, as much as they will bend, keeping the neck extended for 30 seconds at a time. This extension enhances the force of vacuum and brings water into the disc spaces. At the same time, because of their front attachment to the spinal ligament, all of the discs will be retracted back into their normal spaces between the vertebrae and away from the nerve roots in the neck.

Another simple procedure to correct this problem is lying on one's back on the very edge of the bed with the head hanging back and down. This posture permits the weight of the head to stretch the non-weight-bearing neck and bend it backward. A few moments of total relaxation in this position will ease the tension in the neck. This is a good posture to generate a type of vacuum in the disc spaces in the neck. After gently bending the head backward so that you can see the floor, raise the head until you see the wall beyond your feet. This procedure may be effective in creating an intermittent vacuum in the vertebral spaces between any two vertebrae. The vacuum draws water into the disc spaces and spreads it to all parts in the neck joints and lubricates their movements. This water is needed for the disc core to re-expand to its natural size, jacking up and separating one vertebra from the other. You could now bend the head from one side to the other. Try to look at the wall and floor of the room, first one side and then the other side. People who begin to suffer from neck 'arthritis' or disc displacement in the neck may wish to test this simple procedure to improve the mobility of their neck joints.

Anginal pain

For more information read the section on cholesterol. In brief and to address the dehydration-produced pains of the body together, anginal pain means water shortage in the body. The common factor in all the conditions labelled as different diseases of the heart and the lungs is an established dehydration.

Headaches

In my personal experience, migraine headaches seem to be brought about by dehydration; excess bed covers that will not permit the body to regulate its temperature during sleep; alcoholic beverages (hangover) initiating a process of cellular dehydration, particularly in the brain; dietary or allergic triggers for histamine release; excess environmental heat without water intake. Basically, migraine seems to be an indicator of critical body temperature regulation at times of heat stress. Dehydration plays a major role in the precipitation of migraine headaches.

The most prudent way of dealing with migraine is its prevention by the regular intake of water. Once migraine breaks the pain barriers, a cascade of chemical reactions will stop the body from further activity. At this time, one has to take pain-relieving medications with copious water. Sufficient cold or iced water may by itself be able to cool the body (and also the brain) from inside, and promote closing of the vascular system everywhere. Excess dilation of the peripheral vessels might well be the basic cause of migraine headache.

Mrs Mavis Butler, a touring Australian Adventist missionary in Silang in the Philippines, has an interesting history. She has for many years suffered from migraine headaches. She would at times be so incapacitated as to become bed-ridden. She came across this book when she was in Silang and started to increase her water intake. She wrote to tell me that she has so improved that she now wants to shout it from the house-tops. Mrs Butler's is another of those human stories that make one wonder how it is possible that we were so ignorant of the importance of water to health that people could suffer from its lack in the body, to the point of wishing to die.

Cancer – an overview

'Our great grandchildren will look back at this period and wonder how we could condemn one third of the population to cancer, when for the last 50 years we've had good evidence that much of this disease could be eradicated.' - **Ross Hulme Hall, Chairman, Dept. Biochemistry, McMaster University**

There is a direct relationship between dehydration – what I perceive as lasting, deep dehydration in the interior of the cells, not the traditionally understood dehydration from the environment around the body cells – and nearly 100 major and minor health problems in the human body. You've already read that obesity and depression are complications of dehydration. In this section, I will try to explain, in simple terms, why cancer is also the outcome of water shortage. To pique your interest and to show that the WaterCure works for cancer, let me begin by sharing with you an e-mail I received from Patrick M. on how his prostate biopsy was cancer-free even when his PSA was high.

I want to thank you - I just got the biopsy result from the biopsy done on my prostate and they showed "absolutely no sign of cancer". My doctor had warned me that my PSA (prostate blood test) was very high and the "free factor" very low – an indication I had cancer. I had been on the WaterCure programme and so was disappointed. I know now that the programme is valid and thank you for your support. I will get even more serious and never give up drinking my 100 oz a day. Regards, Patrick

Let us now see why water is a preventive medication against cancer.

What is cancer, and why does it eventually kill?

Cancer is a 'selfish', invasive type of tissue that develops within an organ of the body. It breaks the natural boundaries of the mother

111

organ and eventually spreads rapidly, disproportionately, and invasively, resulting in fatal disruption of normal body functions, to the point of exhaustion and death. What is the difference between cancer cells and other ordinary cells in the same organ?

The natural characteristics of cancer cells:
Primitive and genetically selfish
Anaerobic – low oxygen needs
Reveal stem cell characteristics in some cell culture media

As the cells in the body mature, they develop sophisticated communication skills. They develop all kinds of receivers and sensors on their membranes. These sensors are needed to coordinate the cell's activity with the rest of the body. They integrate the cell and its specialized activity into the larger scheme of body physiology. One class of sensors on the cell membrane controls the boundaries up to which the cell will grow and not beyond. These sensors feel the presence of the other cells in their proximity. They maintain a safe distance from neighbouring cells via the messaging system between the membrane receptors and the DNA mechanisms of the cell that control its growth and reproduction.

The role of histamine in the immune system
The defence system of the body depends on the precise action of its white cells. There are six different types of white cells - neutrophils, eosinophils, basophils, monocytes, lymphocytes and plasma cells. The lymphocytic cells normally constitute about 30 per cent of all white cells in the body. Most white cells, much like constantly cruising police cars, leave the blood circulation and enter into various tissues to bolster the state of the local defence system; they then re-enter the blood circulation via the lymphatic system. Some white cells become fixed local protective shields until used and then replaced.

Lymphocytes are mostly responsible for the manufacture of antibodies to offending agents, whereas the other white cells engage in 'eating and digesting' dead and dying cells, as well as intruding elements. The antibodies from the lymphocytic line of defence attach themselves to the element that is recognized as an outsider – bacteria, viruses, parasites – and not only neutralize their toxicity but also label them for scavenging cells to devour and digest.

Like mast cells that get programmed in the lymphatic patches, the lymphocytes that need to engage in antibody formation also get programmed in the thymus gland, possibly in the liver, and definitely in the bone marrow. The ones schooled in the thymus gland are called T-cells; those from the bone marrow, B-cells. T-cell lymphocytes are divided into three subsets – helper-T-cells, cytotoxic or killer-T-cells, and suppressor-T-cells. Among them, these T-cells regulate the immune system via the chemical agents they produce, such as the interleukins (interleukin-2 to inellcukin-6), interferon and stimulant factor for growth of the other white cells.

Histamine is also a major regulator of the complex roles of the white cells in the operation of the immune activity when there is a genuine call on the immune system. However, the system need not, and indeed must not, become activated by histamine when it engages in the drought-management programmes of the body. This is how it works.

The immune system is suppressed by histamine in the bone marrow, where all the immune activity of the body originates. Suppressor T-cells are highly responsive to the action of histamine – and as it happens, there are twice as many suppressor cells as helper cells permanently residing in the bone marrow. Thus, histamine puts a tight lock on the bone marrow activity through its strong influence on the larger local population of suppressor T-cells. This is how histamine prevents flare-ups of the immune system at its bone marrow origin when it gets engaged in the drought-management programmes of the body.

This information has vast ramifications. Not only does it apply to the prevention of diseases such as cancer and the autoimmune disorders, but it also highlights how, gradually and yet surely, short-changing the body from the water it must receive daily is invitation to disaster. My book *Water Cures: Drugs Kill* has shown that water can reverse more than 90 major and minor health problems.

Breast cancer

If ever a cancer story were to make you think twice about trusting the mainstream medical establishment and its offers of chemotherapy, radiation and surgery, it is the firsthand experience of Lorraine Day MD ('No relation!' – Phillip), a renowned orthopaedic surgeon herself with many years of teaching hospital experience. For 15 years she was on the faculty of the University of California, San Francisco, School of Medicine – considered among the top three medical schools in America. She was an associate professor, vice chairman of the Department of Orthopaedic Surgery and chief of orthopaedic surgery at San Francisco General Hospital itself, where she was involved in the training of thousands of doctors. She compares her daily routine when she was at S.F. General with the wartime field hospital portrayed in the TV series M.A.S.H.

Dr. Day was a frequent lecturer at many top medical institutions in America and Europe, including the Massachusetts Medical Society and the Royal Society of Medicine in London, England – both very prestigious centres of thought. In short, she was considered one of mainstream medicine's most highly qualified physicians, qualified enough to mould the minds of emerging doctors. At this point in her life, and at the peak of her dizzying medical achievements, the Creator enrolled her in His own medical school and threw her into the deep waters of the unknown as He had with me a number of years before. Dr. Day developed a very fast-growing breast cancer in 1992.

She immediately knew that what knowledge she had about cancer was not enough, and that the prevalent treatments she had used for her patients were not what she wanted for herself. As she correctly says, doctors are more afraid of cancer than other diseases. They know the treatments they offer others do not work. Within days she realized she would die soon. Her initial small tumour, protruding through the middle of her chest from her left breast, grew to the size of a large orange in about three weeks. She could not rely on her medical colleagues at her own university to deal with her medical emergency. Based on her obvious sanity and the information she had gathered, she did not wish to be another victim of the commerce-protected cancer treatment protocol. She states, *"I refused chemotherapy, radiation and mutilating surgery because, as a medical doctor with years of experience, I saw thousands of cancer patients die, not from their cancer, but from the painful, maiming, destructive treatments we doctors give them."*

She stopped practising medicine and became a student of 'alternative medicine'. She started reading copiously about the natural treatment procedures offered by alternative medicine practitioners. She changed her lifestyle and started to look into nutrition for answers to her problem. The cancer was growing and would soon begin to break her skin and ulcerate, exposing her to the additional problems of infection. She found a surgeon to only remove the external tumor and did nothing about its fast-growing secondaries in the glands in her armpit, in the space above her collarbone, in her nose, and elsewhere – and no chemotherapy and no radiation.

The cancer came back with a vengeance and grew at rapid rates all over again despite her new diet. She became so weak that she could hardly walk and was nursed in her bed. At these final stages of her life, when the archangel was getting ready to accompany her to the

Pearly Gates – and she knew it, too – as if God wanted to make an ignorance-shattering point in medicine and set her up as another of His medical messengers, someone gave her a copy of my book *Your Body's Many Cries for Water*. All at once she realized the information in the book was speaking to her problem and she began to drink water as if there were no tomorrow.

She realized the coffee she had been drinking all those years between operations, in place of water her body wanted, had done the damage and set her up for the development of the cancer she was now facing. The addition of water to Dr. Day's daily diet gave the archangel his marching orders and she started feeling better every day. It took about eight months for her to recover completely and become cancer-free. She has been cancer-free for the past ten years. You can visit her website at www.drday.com.

She now speaks at different conferences for the public, as well as to those from the medical establishment who are exercising intelligence and do not wish to hurt people now that a simpler alternative treatment protocol for cancer is available. Medical professionals whose family members develop cancer, or who have it themselves, seek her newly gained wisdom. She has adopted my book *Your Body's Many Cries for Water* as one of her teaching tools.

In March 2003 we met for the first time at a medical conference in Phoenix, Arizona. I asked her what made her think water played a pivotal role in the treatment of her cancer, when she is expanding her recommendations to include many different things. Her answer revealed the maturity of a true scientist. She told me she was doing all the other things before she incorporated water into her protocol, but without water they did not work. It was water that truly made the difference. Using all the other steps in her current recommendation, and no water, she was sinking fast and became immobile and was forced to stay mostly in bed. She has stated more than once: "Dr.

116

Batmanghelidj's book, Your Body's Many Cries for Water, was critical in my recovery. I could not have gotten well without that addition to my plan."

What could possibly speed cancer growth in the breast to the point that a tumour could expand to the size of a grapefruit, as in the case of Dr. Day? If I were to bet on any element in the chain of chemical events associated with dehydration, it would be increased prolactin production. Prolactin is one of the stress hormones of the body and also one of the hormones driving the gland tissue in the breast to produce milk. Its increased production in stress is designed to compensate for the possible negative effect of dehydration on milk production. It is interesting to note that even birds have similar secretory glands in the back of their mouths, from which a kind of 'milk' is squirted into the mouth of their chicks while in the nest. Milk, apart from being a source of energy and primary raw materials, also transfers the immunoglobulins of the mother to the child during the time that the child's immune system is not fully developed.

Prostate cancer

The prostate gland has an enzyme system that is responsive to increased acidity in its environment. Once the enzyme acid phosphatase gets activated, it begins to promote protein formation and the enlargement of the tissues around it. Thus, persistent dehydration and low acid clearance from the body are the primers for the hypertrophy of the prostate gland. Correcting dehydration and making the body alkaline can reverse the process. Here is one example. Please note that the process will also alleviate other problems.

Dear Dr. B,

I recently read your book Your Body's Many Cries for Water and I have seriously been following your advice since the first of January, drinking 8-10 glasses of water per day.

Three things have happened to me physically since I started following your advice. First the prostate problems that I have had for more than eight years seem to be getting much, much better. As you can see, I live in a high, dry place. Prior to your book I could not sleep through the night because of the dryness in my nose and mouth. Now, I have no problems. Finally, the fungus that I have had under my toenails since the Korean War is gone!

I know many more important things have been reported to you, but these were important to me. I appreciate all the work you're doing.

Regards, R. D. B.

Note: The fungus disappeared because R.D.B.'s immune system was released from its inhibited state. This enabled it to deal with the fungus as well as any early cancer transformation in the prostate tissue itself.

Skin cancer

For the treatment of skin cancers, repeated bathing and hot-water massage of the cancer tissue may prove very effective. You need to bring more circulation to the base of skin to fight the cancer cells. Hot water will help. I got to know a Princeton professor who told me about his experience with an extensive ulcerating melanoma of his back. After he could not get any relief from his treatments in one of the teaching hospitals in Philadelphia, he instinctively decided to stay in his bathtub for two hours a day and soak his back with warm water. He would sometimes use some mineral salts in the water. He cured his own cancer in this way.

I met a lady at my first lecture - Cancer: Another Cry for Water - at the Cancer Control Society conference in San Diego in 1994. She had a very large cancer at the back of her left hand. She had decided to attend one of the famous clinics in California that use lifestyle and nutrition changes to treat disease. She wanted to know my opinion and if she could do anything more to get rid of her cancer.

I told her to drink water and to soak her hand in warm water as often as she could daily. The institution she attended did not advocate water consumption. Its staff believed only in 'juicing' the body. I ran into this woman again in 2002, at the same conference in Los Angeles. She told me her cancer had healed very rapidly after she used water internally as well as bathing her hand in warm water. Here is the why of it.

Skin dehydration

The structure of skin is made up of several layers. There is an external, compacted dying-cells layer that is exposed to the elements outside the body. Immediately beneath this compacted layer is the layer of vibrantly lively skin cells that constantly grow and replace the external layer, which peels off and gets scraped because of friction. Then, under the actively growing layer, is a layer of fatty deposits that act as a shock-absorber and heat- and cold-insulator for the structures beneath it, such as muscle tissue and superficial bones. Two layers of capillary circulation serve the skin. One layer is located between the skin layer and fat under it. Another mesh of capillaries is found under the fat layer, just over the muscle tissue. These two meshworks are interconnected by branches that traverse the fatty layer.

When we are young and the cells of the body are well hydrated, blood circulation in the outermost mesh of capillaries serves the skin, because the body has enough water reserves to afford its constant loss to the atmosphere – hence the rosy colour of the skin in the young. As we age and our perception of thirst becomes less acute, permitting the body to become unintentionally dehydrated, the outer capillary bed is closed down more and more. The sub-fatty layer of capillaries provides some blood circulation to the skin cells, but hardly enough to compensate for the constant loss of water from the skin – hence the grey, furrowed, dehydrated skin in the elderly.

Proper hydration by mouth – including the restoration of the salt and mineral reserves of the body – opens up the capillary circulation in the sub-skin layer. The heat from hot-water immersion of the skin stimulates the nerve endings in the area. They cause the sub-skin capillary bed to open up and supply the water needed for perspiration and sweating to cool the body. In the process, some toxic waste is also excreted through the sweat glands.

Thus, as a treatment protocol for skin cancers, hot water serves a dual purpose. First, the skin sensors also let the brain know that water is available and that its rationing programs – which shut down surface circulation to the skin in the first place – need not be strictly executed. Second, the heat supplied by water causes the capillary bed to open up and bring more water, oxygen, raw materials and energized immune cells to the base of the cancerous growth in the skin – a natural and effective treatment protocol for superficial cancers.

Note: To deal with cancer tissue, the body has to bring more circulation to the area. Since the insufficiency of microcirculation and low oxygen flow are the primary trigger mechanisms for cancer transformation of local cells, correction of the problem is the first step toward repairing the damage. Toward this end, the local vascular bed of capillaries will need to expand and new blood vessels be formed. The process is known as angiogenesis. Commercial medicine, always looking for a moneymaking angle, has presented the body's natural defence mechanism of forming more blood vessels to fight disease as something the cancer cells do to grow. They have tried to produce chemicals to prevent angiogenesis with results that are, as far as I have heard, catastrophic. Such treatments should be avoided. Hydrate and make the body alkaline to fully activate its defence systems. Let the body deal with the problem naturally and without commercial interference.

Cancer: what you can do

'Let us go to the ignorant savage, consider his way of eating and be wise.' – **Harvard Professor Ernest Hooten**

Phillip Day: For twenty-five years I have studied cancer and the medical establishment's inability to reverse the disease. My conclusions? Cancer is the judgement bar of lifestyle. Cancer is, at the same time, the most feared and politically directed illness we have. The reason medicine has so far failed to relieve society of this scourge is because cancer is a metabolic problem and doctors are not trained in nutrition or water science. My bestselling book, *Cancer Why We're Still Dying to Know the Truth,* details the colossal medical fraud that is practised in the name of cancer science. Here now, let me summarise the straight-forward diet, hydration and lifestyle program with Dr B's comments included that has seen thousands worldwide clear their condition.

Dietary changes:

Change to a low GI anti-candida diet to restrict high glucose-yielding foods. Sugar feeds cancer. Grains are out, along with potatoes and other high-efficiency energy foods. The usual mix of alcohol and carbonated soft drinks so endemic in our society is also out. Drink water!! What you end up with is small amounts of white meat if you wish (ensure organic) and cold-caught fish, and the awesome pantheon of complex carb greens and other cancer-fighting foods for the duration of your condition. See my book to find out what the experts recommend to alkalise the body and ensure a high rate of enzymes into the system. Veggie juicing is great. Avoid fruit juice (acid plus fructose).

Dr Batmanghelidj: Green is good for you. Chlorophyll contains much magnesium, in the same way haemoglobin contains much iron. They are both oxygen carriers. Chlorophyll has the effect of making

121

the body alkaline. Green vegetables contain many vital elements needed to sustain life – vitamins, minerals, proteins, essential fats, antioxidants and phytochemicals. If you get uncomfortable eating bulky vegetables, you can always juice them.

Hydrate and salt!

Phillip Day: Cancer is an anaerobic, acid-rich, fermentation environment which hosts yeast and fungal overgrowths. Like any system, the cancer system can be wrecked. Dr B has given us all the reasons to hydrate, not only with water, but with high water-content, high-fibre, living whole organic plant dietary to accomplish this. Washing out the acid is *de rigeur* for cancer recovery. Salt, in the form of sodium bicarbonate, is used by oncologist Dr Tullio Simoncini, to destroy tumours in as little as ten days.[14] *Fungi and parasites hate salt.* I favour Himalayan salt and recommend it in the ratios advocated by Dr Batmanghelidj: Half a teaspoon to a teaspoon per ten glasses of water, according to bodyweight.

Supplement!

Phillip Day: Take a comprehensive liquid mineral supplement (I favour Neways' Maximol – a highly bioavailable colloidal liquid mineral mix [15]). Vitamin C complex (not just ascorbic acid). Vitamin D plus sunshine, Vitamins A & E in their emulsified form (not from the cornershop) and Vitamin B17 in the form of apricot kernels and/or B17 tablets (www.cytopharmaexpress.com). Some people who cannot afford supplements rely on diet alone and, depending on the cancer and state of their immune system, many make it. Find out the scientific rationale behind fish oils, selenium and CoQ 10. Drink Essiac tea. Spread your supplementation throughout the day so you're washing the body with nutrients. Yeast and fungi figure prominently with most cancers, so incorporate garlic (allicin), wormwood, astragalus,

---

[14] www.cancerfungus.com
[15] www.neways.com

echinacea, charcoal, peppermint, cinnamon and ginger into your re-birth repertoire.[16]

Dr Batmanghelidj: A balance of minerals in the diet is crucial to preventing cancer. It becomes even more critical for the treatment of cancers. You need salt to expand the volume of blood in circulation so that it stays dilute and reaches all the nooks and crannies of the body. Salt will also help make the inside of the cells of the body alkaline, essential for preventing and treating cancer. The other mineral components of unrefined [organic] salt – calcium, magnesium, potassium, selenium, zinc and up to 80 other trace elements – expand the water content of the cell interior and make it alkaline. Thus, unrefined sea salt, or unrefined salt from land deposits must be used instead of regular table salt that has been stripped of its vitally important companion minerals.

Exercise!

Phillip Day: The last thing a cancer patient is told to do by his oncologist is exercise, yet exercise galvanises the metabolism, drives down insulin levels, drags large amounts of oxygen into the body, boosts immunity and pumps the lymphatic system. A more effective way to destroy the fermentation environment and promote proper oxygenation you cannot imagine. Exercising for the purposes of cancer *is not walking*, it's getting the heart-rate up to around 65-70% of your maximum (which is 220 minus your age) for around 40-60 minutes a day. Simply put, turn yourself into the best condition of your life and one of the side-effects will be no more cancer. If you are disabled or cannot move well, the hunt is on for other ways to raise your heart rate, while stationary cycling, hill-climbing, stair-climbing and all those wondrous gismos in the gym are all good for the remainder.

---

[16] For full details, see my book, *Cancer: Why We're Still Dying to Know the Truth*, available at www.credence.org

Dr Batmanghelidj: Exercise is one of the physiological pedestals on which life stands. It helps blood circulate into all corners of the body, hydrate and oxygenate each region and preserve local health. Proper regional hydration and oxygenation of tissues are sure steps to cancer prevention. Exercise is vital for efficient lymphatic flow back to the heart. Muscle contraction exerts pumping pressure and forces the lymph to flow in the lymphatic vessels upward and onward to reach the heart and get mixed with blood to be circulated again. Exercise will direct the body physiology toward conservation of tryptophan and the other essential amino acids, vital for prevention of cancer.

Sunlight, and its subset of light systems, reaches and stimulates the special sensors on the skin of the face and the forehead, as well as the light sensors of the eye. These energy fields of light programme and set the biological clock of the body to naturally integrate the hormonal secretion of its glands. Sunlight is a healing energy. It helps correct osteoporosis and the soft-bone complications of rickets in children. Sunlight converts cholesterol to vitamin D and encourages storage of ATP energy in the calcium deposits within the cells of the body - a vital step in boosting the immune activity of the body.

Music: Masaru Emoto, MD, an outstanding Japanese scientist, has introduced a new topic into the science of medicine. He has discovered that water is influenced both by what it 'hears' and by the toxins that pollute it. Emoto has demonstrated this phenomenon by influencing water with sound, or taking water from sources that already contain toxins, and then freezing that water until it forms ice crystals. Classical and harmonious music produces clear, smooth ice crystals. Loud heavy-metal music produces abnormal or deformed crystals. The ice from water that contains toxins, such as dioxin, produces abnormal and deformed ice crystals. Even kind or unkind words such as 'thank you' or 'devil' written on the glass influence the shape and texture of the ice crystals.

"*Love and thankfulness show the most beautiful crystals in the world,*" Emoto reports. Mozart, Bach, and Chopin produced different variations on 'happy ice crystals'. These experiments leave no room for doubt that water reacts to what it hears. Remember, the body is about 75 per cent water; the influence of harmonious sound can thus translate into the inner harmony of our body with the powers of nature in us, exerting a strong healing influence. Happiness-generating music should be used in the treatment protocol of any disease, particularly as an effective natural process in cancer treatment.

Note: There is a belief among some scientists that water retains the memory of its past encounters. Dr. Benveniste of INSERM in France is the person who, based on some experiments in his laboratory, first announced the discovery, which was later discredited by *Nature* in its July 28, 1988 publication. In November of 1989 I wrote to Dr. Benveniste and showed him where his experiment was faulty and why his conclusions were erroneous. You could read my published letter among the scientific articles at www.watercure.com. Dr. Emoto's findings about the influence of sound on water may be used wrongly to resurrect Dr. Benveniste's erroneous claims. At a conference in Munich in October of 2003 where Dr. Emoto and I were speakers, I asked him if the ice with 'influenced' shapes melt and that water is frozen again, does it retain the memory of what had influenced it the first time, and does it reproduce the modified shape? His reply was, "*It does not.*" I believe it is incorrect to claim water retains the memory of its past encounters.

Diabetes (an overview)

'It's supposed to be a secret but I'll tell you anyway. We doctors do nothing. We only help and encourage the doctor within.'
- Albert Schweitzer MD

Diabetes seems to be the end result of water deficiency in the brain, to the point that the brain's neurotransmitter systems, particularly the system that is regulated by the neurotransmitter serotonin, are affected. It is within the automatic design of the brain to peg up the glucose threshold so that it can maintain its own volume and energy requirements when there is a water shortage in the body. When there is a gradually establishing chronic dehydration in the body, the brain has to depend more on glucose as a source of energy. The brain needs more glucose for its energy value and its metabolic conversion to water. Under the urgent circumstances produced by stress, up to 85 per cent of the supplemental energy requirement by the brain is provided by sugar alone. This is why stressed people resort to eating sweet food. While all the other cells need to be influenced by insulin to take up glucose through their cell walls, the brain does not depend on insulin to carry sugar across its cell membranes.

It seems to be in the natural design of the brain to steer the physiological mechanisms in the direction of higher glucose levels in the body when there is persistent dehydration that would damage the brain more than it could recover from. The brain resuscitates itself in the same way that a doctor resuscitates a patient – with intravenous fluid containing sugar and salt. The main problem stems from one very important factor – the salt metabolism (both sodium and potassium) of the body also becomes negatively affected when there is water deficiency in the body. This condition should be treated with an increase in water intake and diet manipulation to provide the necessary minerals and amino acid balance for tissue repair – including brain tissue requirements.

126

It has been shown that the brain amino acid balance for tryptophan is affected in diabetic rats. There seems to be a much lower level of this amino acid in the brain when diabetes exists. Tryptophan in turn regulates the salt intake of the body. Salt is responsible for regulating water-volume content outside the cells of the body. When there is tryptophan deficiency in the body, there is also a total body-salt shortage. With lower salt retention as a result of tryptophan deficiency, the responsibility for holding water in the body and outside the cells falls onto the sugar content in the blood. To do its new job and compensate for the lower salt, the sugar content rises. The way this happens is so simple it is almost unbelievable.

One of histamine's deputies, which becomes increasingly active in water-distribution systems, is prostaglandin E. This chemical inhibits the insulin-making cells in the pancreas, preventing them from making and secreting insulin. When insulin is not adequately secreted, the main body cells do not receive sufficient sugar and some amino acids. Potassium stays outside the cells, and the water that accompanies potassium does not enter the cells, either. In this way, the cells of the body are forced to forgo their right to water and some amino acids, and they gradually become damaged. This is how diabetes becomes the cause of many associated disease conditions.

Diabetes is a good example of next-generation damage that is caused by dehydration. Whereas the onset of dehydration-induced diabetes is normally seen in the elderly and is often reversible, the more structurally serious and irreversible variety of the disease is seen in younger people. The juvenile variety of diabetes needs to be treated carefully before it becomes a totally irreversible type of diabetes and permanent structural damage takes place. Basically the cause is the same in children as in adults, except that in adults there is more 'reserve in the system'. In children, the process of physical growth strains the system much more quickly. Children are constantly dehydrated, and their amino acid pool is in a state of constant fluctuation.

At the moment, there seems to be total reliance on the belief that genetic dictation is what promotes the occurrence of diabetes, particularly in the young. One important fact to remember is that the DNA structure is held together by proteins that also obey the many dictates of water as their ultimate regulator. Water is the common factor for all protein functions in the body, including the DNA-manufacturing system. Accordingly, the associated genetic marker in diabetes may not be a dictating factor for disease production; rather, it may be the indicator of a deep-rooted, dehydration-caused damage that has also affected the DNA recording system – a passive outcome.

Pancreas: the failed organ in diabetes

The pancreas, where insulin is made, is an organ that is directly involved in the regulation of the balance between the water compartments of the body. The water volume held inside each cell is regulated and held by the amount of potassium that is forced into the cell. Insulin is a very effective agent for forcing potassium (and amino acids) inside the cells. If potassium stays outside the cells and in circulation, at a certain threshold it can produce irregular heartbeats and, often, a sudden heart seizure and stopping of the heart's rhythmic contractions. In effect, therefore, insulin regulates water volume inside the cell. It manages this responsibility by pushing potassium and sugar into the cell that has insulin-sensitive gates of entry on its outer membrane.

The pancreas has another equally important responsibility. It has to collect water from some of its cells, mix it with manufactured bicarbonate and pancreatic enzymes, and secrete the mixture into the intestine to neutralize the acid that is poured into the intestine from the stomach and begin the next phase of digestion of food. The mixture is known as *watery bicarbonate solution.*

The role of the pancreas in water rationing

If water is in short supply, the watery bicarbonate solution secreted into the intestine cells may not be enough to neutralize all the acid that enters the intestine to begin the cycle of food digestion. Consequently, one or the other process has to be halted. Either the acid has to stop coming into the intestine, or water has to be delivered to the pancreas in a sufficient amount for the pancreas to perform at least one of its functions. A commensurate reduction of insulin secretion stops the entry of water and nutrients into the peripheral cells in the rest of the body that depend on the presence of insulin for their feeding process. By this process, more water will be available in the circulating blood to be delivered to the pancreas to make its watery bicarbonate solution. When the insulin-stimulated gates are not efficient in delivering water and raw materials into the cells, they begin to wither and die. This is the mechanism behind the degenerative process associated with diabetes.

In dyspeptic cases, acid will continue to build up in the stomach. The ring muscle between the stomach and the intestine will close the gap, and nothing will enter the intestine. The more the stomach contracts to push its load into the intestine, the tighter the ring will contract. Only a fraction of the load is let out. Over time, ulcerations in the ring area are produced. In this situation, the full acid load does not enter into the intestine, and less demand is placed on the pancreas for secretion of its watery bicarbonate solution.

In diabetes, the action of insulin in pushing water into the cells is stopped. This is done simply by a two-step process: The first step, a reversible one, is to prevent insulin secretion from the cells that manufacture it. This type of diabetes is called insulin-independent diabetes. The pancreas has the ability to secrete insulin. A second and much more drastic, ruthless and irreversible way is to destroy the insulin-making cells. The process involves the destruction of their nuclei. Enough of their DNA/RNA system is dismembered to make them ineffective as insulin producers. This kind of diabetes is known as insulin-dependent or type I diabetes.

Insulin-independent diabetes (type 2)

This form of diabetes is often reversible. When the insulin-secreting cells are temporarily inhibited by prostaglandin E, certain outside agents can override this and get insulin released. The knowledge of this process of insulin release has been used in devising a simpler treatment procedure than insulin injections. The agents that release insulin are given in tablet form, usually one tablet once a day.

These tablets are normally given to elderly diabetics and not to young ones. There are side-effects to these tablets, including abnormalities in blood cell count and blood cell composition, jaundice, gastro-intestinal symptoms, liver-function problems and skin rashes. Hypoglycaemic coma is also a complication of overdose of these tablets, often the result of forgetful repeat of medication. The use of these drugs is dangerous in liver disease and kidney-function irregularities or deficiency.

In insulin-independent diabetes, a regular daily adjustment of water intake to no less than two quarts, and some increased salt intake, is the best treatment. In this form of diabetes, when the body makes some insulin but does not release it because of the effect of prostaglandin E, water intake and adjustment of diet and minerals often will reverse the situation, and the need for higher blood sugar will subside.

Insulin-dependent diabetes (type 1)

Diabetes can become permanently established when there is DNA/RNA damage. In this type of diabetes, the ability to manufacture insulin is lost. If prostaglandin E remains in general circulation long enough, it activates the hormone interleukin-6. This chemical works its way into the nucleus of insulin-producing cells and gradually dismembers the DNA/RNA scaffolding of the nucleus, decreasing its size and reducing its ability to function. Thus water deficiency, if uncorrected for a long time, can in many people cause damage – sometimes permanent – to their insulin-producing cells.

Subsequently, even more damage to the diabetic body can occur. Some organs begin to suffer and become useless. A leg can shrink and become gangrenous if not amputated; cysts can form in the brain; eyes can become blind.

Diabetes in children

In children, the process is the same, except it begins at a much earlier age until it becomes an 'autoimmune' disease. That is to say, the insulin-producing cells are destroyed to avoid the need for constant control of their activity. The body of a child has much less water reserve than that of a grown person. It seems logical to assume that the gap between the inhibition of insulin release and the threshold of insulin cell destruction must also be less wide. Adding to this problem is the fact that a growing body is always dehydrated. Every cell in the soft tissues needs about 75 per cent of its volume to be water to function within the norms of the human body.

When the body is growing under the influence of growth hormone as well as other hormones, and the effect of histamine with its food and water-supply regulation, a form of stress is constantly experienced. This stimulates the thirst sensation and the body will demand water. Plain water should be given, although some parents force their own habits of drinking sodas, tea or juices on their children.

Nothing – but nothing – can substitute for water to satisfy the water needs of the body. It is true that other drinks contain some water but they do not affect the body in the same way as water itself. The vitamins contained in fresh fruit juices are essential for the body. Still, too much of any juice – particularly orange and grapefruit juice – can be harmful. Juices can increase the acidity of the intestine and then the body. Their high potassium content can drastically increase the activation and presence of histamine. This will signal undue stress to the body and a crisis water-rationing state will develop.

The physical growth of the body of a child is an adaptive response to the stresses and demands placed on it. It grows as a result of this stress and histamine's activities are an essential part of the process.

Phillip Day: Type-2 diabetes is an acidic, anaerobic (oxygen-poor) sugar-rich system almost always contaminated with candida. Adopting a low GI anti-candida diet along with hydration, unrefined salt, minerals and progressive exercising is known to help the cells regain their sensitivity to insulin in type-2 diabetics. Governor Mike Huckabee, erstwhile 2008 US presidential hopeful, reversed his diabetes using the type of system expounded in my book, *The ABC's of Disease.* I am completely of the opinion that dehydration is at the heart of the diabetes phenomenon.

Constipation

'Most problems don't exist until a government agency is created to solve them.' – **Kirk Kirkpatrick**

Dr Batmanghelidj: The intestinal tract uses much water to break down solid foods. It has to liquefy the dissolvable components of solid foods to extract their essential elements. Whatever can be dissolved is then absorbed into the blood circulation and transferred to the liver for processing. The refuse that cannot be further broken down is then passed on through the various segments of the gut and gradually compacted for elimination.

Depending on the adequate availability of free water in the body, the refuse will carry with it some of the water that was used to liquefy the food. What water it can carry with it will act as a lubricant to help the refuse move through the large intestine. The last segments of the small intestine and most of the large intestine are under the direction of the water regulators to re-absorb as much of the water in the refuse as might be needed by the other parts of the body. The more the body is in need of water, the more there is a determined effort to re-absorb the water available in the intestine. This process puts a drastic squeeze on the refuse to separate its water content and make it available for re-absorption by the mucosa or lining membranes of the large intestine.

The more the body is dehydrated, the slower the motility of the lower intestines in order to allow time for re-absorption of the water content of the refuse. This process of preventing water loss is another of the body's water-preservation mechanisms. One part of the body where water loss is prevented in times of drought management is in the large intestine, through adjustment of the consistency and the rate of flow of the excrements. When the passage of refuse from the large intestine is slowed down, the mucosa absorb the water and the faeces become hard and not fluid enough to flow. The act of expulsion of

133

solid faeces becomes difficult. To prevent this process from taking place, added intake of water and some fibres that hold the water better seems to be the only natural solution to constipation. Remember that haemorrhoids, diverticulitis and polyp formation are common occurrences with chronic constipation. Chronic dehydration and its consequential constipation are primers for cancer formation in the large intestine and the rectum.

Re-absorption of water in the digestive tract also involves the regulating valve between the last part of the small intestine and the first part of the large intestine, known as the ileocecal valve. The valve shuts down and allows the small intestine time to get as much water as possible out of the as-yet-unformed refuse. At certain levels of dehydration, the closing of the valve may become too forceful and may cause spasm. This spasm will translate into pain in the lower right side of the abdomen. This pain can be mistaken for a possible inflammation of the appendix, which is served by the same sensory nerves. In women, this same pain could be mis-diagnosed as either ovarian pain or uterine pain, which can cause anxiety and result in expensive, complicated investigations. Let me give you an example.

Joy is one of my assistants at Global Health Solutions. For the past few months, she was suffering from an uncomfortable pain in the area of her appendix – the lower right side of her abdomen. She was advised by her doctor to have a laparoscopy to see what was causing her pain. A laparoscopy is a visual examination inside the abdomen and involves inserting a small viewing instrument into the abdominal cavity through a small incision in the wall of the abdomen. The examination produced minimal findings – nothing that would explain her pain. She was given some painkillers but the problem did not disappear and continued to bother her more and more. Joy had become more concerned and had further scanning tests. While waiting for the results, she came to me for consultation about some office work. I notice that she was in pain and asked her about it.

I had seen this type of pain before and had relieved it with water. I had used water as a diagnostic test to differentiate between genuine appendicitis pain and dehydration pain that mimics appendicitis. I had written about it in my editorial article, reporting my new method of treating peptic ulcer disease in the June 1983 issue of the *Journal of Clinical Gastroenterology*. I asked Joy to drink a glass of water. Her pain diminished within minutes. The pain disappeared completely when she drank the second glass of water. It had not come back in days. She increased her daily water intake to successfully avoid the pain. Women with pain in their lower abdomen, who have been diagnosed with pain-producing ovarian cysts, inflammation of the fallopian tubes or even fibroids, should test the authenticity of their diagnosis with one or two glasses of water. It may well be that they are only thirsty and their bodies are only crying for water in that particular region.

Autoimmune diseases

Many degenerative conditions that we do not understand are labelled 'autoimmune diseases'. It literally means the body is attacking itself without a good cause – at least a cause that should be clear to us in medicine. And since we have never understood dehydration to be a disease-producing state of body physiology, we have never come across a simple and natural solution to this category of conditions – at least until now.

I studied one of these conditions, which has received the label of lupus, and published my findings in the book *ABC of Asthma, Allergies and Lupus*. I explained why I believe autoimmune diseases should be viewed as conditions produced by persistent unintentional dehydration and its metabolic complications.

In dehydration, through the use of some essential elements as antioxidants to neutralize toxic waste that cannot be excreted because of low urine production, there comes a time when certain vital elements become scarce within the body reserves. However, some of the less vital components of the body have these elements in their assimilated forms. These tissues need to give up some of their precious elements for use in other parts of the body. The whole process is based on priorities and the importance of the elements that are scarce. Under these circumstances and in this category of conditions, the body is forced into a cannibalistic state of physiology. Such cannibalism can cause autoimmune diseases, such as lupus.

The chemical controllers in the body begin to break down certain tissues to compensate for the missing elements the body needs – especially in the brain. The body always puts the brain first. For example, when the insulin-producing cells of the pancreas are fragmented and destroyed, not only will the ensuing diabetes increase the level of sugar in circulation for the brain to use, but the process will also dehydrate the other tissues of the body and make their water content available for the needs of the brain and the nervous system. There are some neurological conditions that follow the same logic, such as multiple sclerosis, Alzheimer's disease, muscular dystrophy and Lou Gehrig's disease or amyotrophic lateral sclerosis (ALS).

Alzheimer's disease

The primary cause of Alzheimer's is chronic dehydration of the body. In my opinion, brain cell dehydration is the primary cause of Alzheimer's disease. Aluminium toxicity is a secondary complication of dehydration in areas of the world with comparatively aluminium-free water (although in the technically advanced Western societies, aluminium sulphate is used in the process of water purification for delivery into the city water supplies!). One of my medical friends took this information to heart and started treating his brother who has Alzheimer's disease by forcing him to take more water every day. His brother has begun to recover his memory, so much so that he can now follow conversation and not frequently repeat himself. The improvement became noticeable in a matter of weeks.

Exercise

The most important factor for survival, after air, water, salt and food, is exercise. Exercise is more important to the health of the individual than sex, entertainment or anything else that might be pleasurable. The following points explain the importance of exercise for better health and pain-free longer life.

- Exercise expands the vascular system in the muscle tissue and prevents hypertension.
- It opens the capillaries in the muscle tissue and, by lowering the resistance to blood flow in the arterial system, causes the blood pressure to drop to normal.
- Exercise builds up muscle mass and prevents the muscles being broken down as fuel.
- Exercise stimulates the activity of fat-burning enzymes for manufacture of the constantly needed energy for muscle activity. When you train, you are, in effect, changing the source of energy for muscle activity. You convert the energy source from sugar that is in circulation to fat that is stored in the muscle itself.
- Exercise makes muscles burn as additional fuel some of the amino acids that would otherwise reach toxic levels in the body. In their more-than-normal levels in the blood—usually reached in an unexercised body—certain branched-chain amino acids cause a drastic destruction and depletion of other vital amino acids. Some of these discarded essential amino acids are constantly needed by the brain to manufacture its neurotransmitters. Two of these essential amino acids are tryptophan and tyrosine. The brain uses tryptophan to make serotonin, melatonin, tryptamine and indoleamine, all of which are antidepressants and regulate sugar level and blood pressure. Tyrosine is used for the manufacture of adrenaline,

noradrenaline and dopamine—vital for the coordination of body physiology when it has to take a physical action, such as fighting, running, playing sports and so on. Excess tyrosine loss from the amino acid reserves of the body is also a primary factor in Parkinson's disease.

- Unexercised muscle gets broken down. As a result of the excretion of muscle parts from the body, some of the reserves of zinc and vitamin B6 also get lost. At a certain stage of this constant depletion of vitamin B6 and zinc, certain mental disorders and neurological complications occur. In effect, this happens in autoimmune diseases, including lupus and muscular dystrophy.

- Exercise makes the muscles hold more water in reserve and prevent increased concentration of blood that would otherwise damage the lining of the blood vessel walls.

- Exercise lowers blood sugar in diabetics and decreases their need for insulin or tablet medications.

- Exercise compels the liver to manufacture sugar from the fat that it stores or the fat that is circulating within the blood.

- Exercise causes an increase in the mobility of the joints in the body. It causes the creation of an intermittent vacuum inside the joint cavities. The force of the vacuum causes suction of water into the cavity. Water in the joint cavity brings dissolved nutrients to the cells inside the cartilage. Increased water content of the cartilage also adds to its lubrication and smoother bone-on-bone gliding movements of the joint.

- Leg muscles act as secondary hearts. By their contractions and relaxations during the time we are upright, the leg muscles overcome the force of gravity. They pump into the venous system the blood that was sent to the legs. Because of the pressure breakers—and one-directional valves in the vein—the blood in the leg veins is pushed upward against gravity by frequent contraction of the leg muscles. This is how the leg muscles act as hearts for the venous system in the body. This is a value to exercise that not many people appreciate. Leg muscles also cause an equally effective flow within the lymphatic system and cause oedema in the legs to disappear.

- Exercise strengthens the bones of the body and helps prevent osteoporosis.
- Exercise increases the production of all vital hormones, enhancing libido and heightening sexual performance.
- One hour of walking will cause the activation of fat-burning enzymes, which remain active for 12 hours. A morning and afternoon walk will keep these enzymes active round the clock and will cause clearance of cholesterol deposits in the arterial system.
- Exercise will enhance the activity of the adrenaline-operated sympathetic nerve system. Adrenaline will also reduce the over-secretion of histamine and, as a result, prevent asthma attacks and allergic reactions—providing the body is fully hydrated.
- Exercise will increase production of endorphins and enkephalins, the natural opiates of the body. They produce the same 'high' that drug addicts try to achieve through their abusive intake.

What are the best forms of exercise?

Exercising the body for endurance is better than exercising it for speed or building excess muscle. In selecting an exercise, you should consider its lifetime value. A long-distance runner will enjoy the exercise value of long-distance runs into old age. A sprinter will not sprint for exercise at a later phase of life.

The best exercise that one can benefit from even to a ripe old age, and without causing damage to the joints, is walking. Other exercises that will increase one's endurance are swimming, golf, skiing, skating, climbing, tennis, squash, cycling, tai chi, dancing and aerobics. In selecting an exercise, one should evaluate its ability to keep the fat-burning enzymes active for longer durations. Outdoor forms of exercise are more beneficial for the body than indoor forms. The body becomes better connected to 'nature'.

Summary

Forty-six reasons why your body needs water every day

1. Without water, nothing lives.
2. Comparative shortage of water first suppresses and eventually kills some aspects of the body.
3. Water is the main source of energy - it is the 'cash flow' of the body.
4. Water generates electrical and magnetic energy inside each and every cell of the body – it provides the power to live.
5. Water is the bonding adhesive in the architectural design of the cell structure.
6. Water prevents DNA damage and makes its repair mechanisms more efficient – less abnormal DNA is made.
7. Water increases greatly the efficiency of the immune system in the bone marrow, where the immune system is formed (all its mechanisms) – including its efficiency against cancer.
8. Water is the main solvent for all foods, vitamins, and minerals. It is used in the breakdown of food into smaller particles and their eventual metabolism and assimilation.
9. Water energizes food, and food particles are then able to supply the body with this energy during digestion. This is why food without water has absolutely no energy value for the body.
10. Water increases the body's rate of absorption of essential substances in food.
11. Water is used to transport all substances inside the body.
12. Water increases the efficiency of red blood cells in collecting oxygen in the lungs.
13. When water reaches a cell, it brings the cell oxygen and takes the waste gases to the lungs for disposal.
14. Water clears toxic waste from different parts of the body and takes it to the liver and kidneys for disposal.

15. Water is the main lubricant in the joint spaces and helps prevents arthritis and back pain.
16. Water is used in the spinal discs to make them 'shock-absorbing water cushions'.
17. Water is the best lubricating laxative and prevents constipation.
18. Water helps reduce the risk of heart attacks and strokes.
19. Water prevents clogging of arteries in the heart and the brain.
20. Water is essential for the body's cooling (sweat) and heating (electrical) systems.
21. Water gives us power and electrical energy for all brain functions, most particularly thinking.
22. Water is directly needed for the efficient manufacture of all neurotransmitters, including serotonin.
23. Water is directly needed for the production of all hormones made by the brain, including melatonin.
24. Water can help prevent attention deficit disorder in children and adults.
25. Water increases efficiency at work; it expands your attention span.
26. Water is a better pick-me-up than any other beverage in the world – and it has no side-effects.
27. Water helps reduce stress, anxiety, and depression.
28. Water restores normal sleep rhythms.
29. Water helps reduce fatigue – it gives us the energy of youth.
30. Water makes the skin smoother and helps decrease the effects of ageing.
31. Water gives lustre and shine to the eyes.
32. Water helps prevent glaucoma.
33. Water normalizes the blood-manufacturing systems in the bone marrow – it helps prevent leukaemia and lymphoma.
34. Water is absolutely vital for making the immune system more efficient in different regions to fight infections and cancer cells where they are formed.
35. Water dilutes the blood and prevents it from clotting during circulation.

36. Water decreases premenstrual pains and hot flushes.
37. Water and heartbeats create the dilution and waves that keep things from sedimenting in the bloodstream.
38. The human body has no stored water to draw on during dehydration. This is why you must drink regularly and throughout the day.
39. Dehydration prevents sex hormone production – one of the primary causes of impotence and loss of libido.
40. Drinking water separates the sensations of thirst and hunger.
41. To lose weight, water is the best way to go – drink water on time and lose weight without much dieting. Also, you will not eat excessively when you feel hungry but are in fact only thirsty for water.
42. Dehydration causes deposits of toxic sediments in the tissue spaces, joints, kidneys, liver, brain, and skin. Water will clear these deposits.
43. Water reduces the incidence of morning sickness in pregnancy.
44. Water integrates mind and body functions. It increases ability to realize goals and purpose.
45. Water helps prevent the loss of memory as we age. It helps reduce the risk of Alzheimer's disease, multiple sclerosis, Parkinson's disease and Lou Gehrig's disease (motor neurone disease).
46. Water helps reverses addictive urges, including those for caffeine, alcohol and some drugs.

Some testimonies

Dear Dr. Batmanghelidj

I had the opportunity of reading some of your publications concerning the significance of adequate hydration and the role of chronic dehydration in the etiology of disease. While perusing this material, I carefully examined many of the references that you had cited, especially those in your paper published in *Anticancer Research* (1987:7:971) and in your subsequent paper in Volume 1 of *Science in Medicine Simplified*.

Every reference that I checked was properly used to support your hypothesis that a paradigm shift from a solute-based to a solvent-based body metabolism is warranted. I conclude, based upon study of your revolutionary concept, that its implementation by health care professionals and by the general public is certain to have an enormous positive impact both on well-being and on health care economics. Accordingly, I will do all that I can to publicise the importance of your findings.

Yours truly,

Barry S. Kendler, Ph.D.

Associate Professor of Biology

Manhattan College

Adjunct Faculty Member

Graduate Nutrition Program

New York Medical College

Migraines

Dear Phillip. When I was in my teens, I suffered many migraines as had my grandmother before me. Nothing the doctors suggested seemed to work and I felt the drugs I was given were very toxic, so discarded them and learned to cope with the migraines. In my twenties, I found of my own volition that drinking water and therefore

145

'flushing through my system' seemed to stop migraines in their tracks. I later found, through reading about dehydration and following on from that, about the benefits of drinking water for migraines. If only the doctor had told me when I was 13 about dehydration, I would have had easier teenage years. I am now 61 and have only had a handful of migraines over the years, all of which I have solved through drinking water and resting until the attack is over. Sylvia B, Devon, UK

Arthritis

Attn: The Honorable F. Batmanghelidj, MD

At 82 years of age I am still in fair shape and only regret I did not have the superb advice of Dr. Batmatighelidj and that of his books, *Your Body's Many Cries for Water* and *Low Back Pain*.

Dr. Batman's reasoning is incisive, his medical knowledge indeed sparkles with wit and brilliant logic. His books are now a treasured possession in my library. I have used his advice for the painful arthritis I have in my hands and back and within two weeks, I have experienced considerable reduction of pain. I sleep better, I have more strength, with greater coordination and relaxation. I see life from a different point of view, where everything seems easier for me to do.

Dr. Batman's books are full of common sense and truthful medical advice. His suggested treatment of disease goes to the roots, the cause of it and anyone who is fortunate enough to read them won't be disappointed with their purchase.

Respectfully,
Laurence A Malone, MD PhD
Dean for Academic Affairs
The Learning Center
Chagrin Falls, Ohio 44023

146

High cholesterol

Dear Dr Batmanghelidj,

This is to say how grateful I am to you for making me a much less worried man. I have suffered from a high cholesterol level since 1982. It was 278 when it was first discovered. I was then in Germany and I was put on such a strict diet that I lost 16 pounds in less than two months and the cholesterol level went down to only 220. I refused to accept to lower it further through medication especially since in Egypt the doctors still believe that this level is not really dangerous by the prevailing standards in our country.

Since I entertain and attend business lunches more than what would be expected even from a diplomat, because of the additional burden of dealing with the media, my cholesterol was always going up to around 260 and back to 220s by putting myself on a very strict diet from time to time. However, it must be noted that it was only outside my home that the diet came crashing down. Otherwise I was strict with myself. In fact, even when I ate outside, I was careful to choose dishes, wherever available, which were not particularly rich in fat.

Last year I was shocked to discover that my blood cholesterol level had shot up to 279. I was lucky to have met you then. When you prescribed ample water (two full glasses) be taken before meals instead of medication that I was just about to submit myself to then, I was very skeptical. All the more so since you did not overemphasize dieting. In two months, and with very little observance of all the old rules which were making my life miserable, my cholesterol went down to 203 for the first time in more than nine years! My weight too was surprisingly also down by about eight pounds and has since been under control. In fact, I feel so good that I am sure that the next time I will be going for a blood test, my cholesterol level will be found to be even lower. So, goodbye to the 'normal' Egyptian standards and welcome to the American new levels of cholesterol without the accompanying sense of deprivation!

Enjoying eating, moderately of course, as I had not been doing for a long time and free from a worry that was always at the back of my mind, I believe I owe you a big THANK YOU.

Yours sincerely,
Minister Mohammed Wahby
Director, Press and Information Bureau
Embassy of the Arab Republic of Egypt

Migraines; IBS

Dear Phillip. I began increasing my water intake after reading Dr Batmanghelidj's book *Your Body's Many Cries for Water* some years ago (bought at one of your talk evenings), and I know that, in addition to changing my diet, I have greatly improved my health and vitality. In particular, migraine headaches, which I used to suffer on a regular basis, became far less frequent and much less severe. I also used to suffer from irritable bowel syndrome and this stopped completely. If I ever feel a headache starting, I drink a couple of glasses of water and it just disappears. At 63, I have plenty of energy and stamina. I particularly notice when I push myself to do an extra strenuous task such as a day's gardening or decorating, I am always surprised how great I feel at the end of day. It is not unknown for me to tackle the ironing or wash the kitchen floor after a day's gardening! Back in the bad old days, I would have run out of steam after a few hours.

I also used to suffer from aching joints, in particular my hips and knees after a night of dancing, but the water intake has definitely sorted out that problem.

I use only rock or sea salt which I grind myself and as I only cook from scratch. I always know how much salt I am having. I steer clear of the chemical-laden table salt. Occasionally, after exercising (I do a lot of walking), I will get cramp and having ruled out that it is not due to dehydration, I deal with this by putting a few crystals of salt on my tongue until they dissolve – taking care to avoid letting it rest too long on the roof of my mouth otherwise it can burn. The cramp soon disappears.

I still work full time in a large, open-plan office and part of my job is being the Display Screen Assessor, which means I have to check that everyone (and that's almost 100 people) are comfortable at their computers, sitting correctly, etc. Many of them used to complain of headaches, neck aches, backaches, etc, and each time I asked how much water they drank. A vast number admitted they drank no water at all(!) so I used to give them a print-out of yours regarding the importance of drinking water and, more importantly, the effects of *not* drinking water. As a result, the water consumption in the office has dramatically increased and the headaches, aches and pains have diminished. A lot of the guys often raise their glasses to me across the office just to let me know they are continuing to drink their water! Kind regards, Jackie B, UK.

Allergies and asthma
Dear Dr. Batmanghelidj:

I am writing to thank you for your kind assistance in treating Jeremy's allergies. As you know, Jeremy is my eight year-old son who suffered for the last 3-4 years with severe allergy symptoms related to allergic rhinitis and asthma.

More recently, he has had significant coryza and coughing which is associated with his asthma. On about the 28th of April 1995, we began a program of rehydration involving his drinking two cups of water before food or exercise and excluding all other fluids. In addition, he consumes a half teaspoon of salt which is added to his food to offset the increased water intake.

Within 3-4 days he showed dramatic improvement; he no longer had severe and excessive mucus production, his coughing had virtually stopped, and his sneezing and other allergy symptoms were totally gone. Therefore we discontinued his Benadryl and Albuterol and continued his hydration program.

Jeremy has been following this program now for approximately four and a half weeks, spending almost four weeks off his medication and is doing quite well. Not only have his symptoms cleared subjectively, but in terms of objective findings, his peak flow volumes have been within normal range. His constant medication-induced drowsiness has disappeared and as a result he is more alert, and his school grades have improved.

Therefore I want to emphasize how effective this treatment has been for Jeremy and I wish you well in sharing this cost-effective and very efficacious program with others.

Once again Dr. Batmanghelidj, I thank you for advising me on the new treatment program of Jeremy's allergies and asthma.

Very truly yours,
Cheryl Brown-Christopher, MD
Lifestyle Medical Center,
Annapolis, Maryland

Migraine; Eyes

Thank you, thank you, and thank you! Thank you for discovering the simplest and greatest miracle cure ever. And thank you for all your years of hard work—no words are adequate. The migraines that destroyed my life for 35 years and my pocketbook are gone-gone-gone-gone, (one of which I would never have dreamed about).

I've been wearing glasses practically all my life (now bifocals) and every year I need stronger glasses—when suddenly two weeks ago my glasses felt awkward somehow—again believing 1 needed a stronger prescription, I went for a check-up. To my shock both eyes got better (upper and lower) and for the first time in my life my glasses are weaker and my eyes stronger.

There have been many other unexpected changes—feel better all over, look better, sleep better, think better, etc. etc. How dehydrated I must have been is unreal—and how dehydrated most everyone is, is truly tragic. I can SEE it in almost all the people I know and meet. Therefore, I talk about WATER constantly and I speak of Dr. Batmanghelidj all the time and my prayer is that the two will soon be known throughout the world, for it is truly God's greatest miracle

cure. Thank you dear Dr. Batmanghelidj—thank you for my life.
Sincerely, M.A.V.

Asthma

Dear Phillip. In 2001 I wrote to a local newspaper here on the New
South Wales Central Coast (Gosford) outlining the way to beat asthma.
That is to say, 'when an attack is imminent the person should drink
water as soon as possible and then put a dab of sea salt on the tip of
the tongue.' I explained the scientific rationale behind these actions.

Three days after the letter was published I received a telephone
call from a local resident named Kurt. Kurt said he had followed the
advice and declared it a 'miracle'. I invited Kurt to my house so I could
explain the 'miracle' further. He was a tall and skinny man with pale
complexion and had other medical problems besides his asthma. He
worked in a large, dusty warehouse as a forklift driver. He still had
some medical problems, except now he had not needed his asthma
medication for five days.

He was still sceptical about vitamins, minerals and a good diet of
fresh vegetables and fruit but would give it a try. I did not see Kurt for
around six months until I was shopping in a local supermarket. I
walked past an employee whom I vaguely recognised from
somewhere. He called out to me, "Peter." I turned. "It's Kurt, I've got a
new job here," he said. I hardly recognised him, he was not so skinny
and definitely not pale anymore. He told me he had listened to the
tape by Dr Batmanghelidj and that I had probably saved his life. I told
him he had probably saved his own life by noting the advice and
taking better care of himself.

In 2001 I went home to Harrogate in Yorkshire, where I helped to
arrange a talk by you. While I was there, my brother-in-law told me he
had just been diagnosed with asthma. I explained the cause of asthma
in about three minutes and he said he would try the sea salt and water.
He called me two days later and said he felt like punching his doctor
on the nose for misleading him. Needless to say, I dissuaded him from
doing so. To date (May 2008) he still has not used an inhaler.

When a person is admitted to hospital with a life-threatening asthma attack, the triage nurse immediately administers oxygen (two litres ph) and calms the patient. The doctor then prescribes intravenous 9% sodium chloride (normal saline) SALTED WATER. This is not a miracle drug but only a doctor can prescribe it and place the cannula. The patient recovers and is released the following day. No one tells the patient to increase their water intake and include salt in their diet. All the asthma, hay fever and lupus sufferers I have encountered tell me that "salt is bad for you!" The UK National Health Service altered its nationwide advertising campaign on salt. Apparently someone had threatened to sue due to bad advice. They now say that "*too much* salt is bad for you". Suffice to say that iatrogenics is still present, even in private hospitals! Peter H, NSW, Australia

Allergies; Heartburn

Thank you for your response. I am a Registered Nurse. I have been trained to think in terms of drugs for a long time. Drug reps are frequent visitors and educators with CEU info. I have also for over 10 years had to take Zantac, Prilosec, Prevacid, Maalox, and Gaviscon on a daily basis. I read the *ABC of Asthma, Allergies, and Lupus* and have to admit I was very skeptical. However, the thing that intrigued me was that there couldn't possibly be any monetary reason to shift someone into a water regimen.

There is just no money in it. I also was getting a bit desperate since, in spite of everything, the medication wasn't working. My doctor was talking of a surgery that would cut nerves in my stomach to reduce the acid production. I am not thrilled with this type of permanent mutilation. I decided to give water a try. It has been nearly two weeks since I decided to give it a try. I have not had any drugs since. As a bonus, my fall allergies have gone away. I am absolutely stunned. I also am sharing it with my patients. I also used to find it very difficult to stick to a diet and have had a lot of trouble losing weight. Not any more. I have lost 5 pounds in 10 days and feel it much easier to say no to snacks. I just wish more people knew about this. Sincerely, D.B.

Sweat; Hot Flushes

I had the book *Your Body's Many Cries For Water* recommended to me and seriously increased my water intake. The benefit I am finding is that my hot flushes and night sweats have dropped dramatically. I am 55 years of age, post-menopausal and was having considerable trouble with both, 24 hours a day. The night sweats have improved so much that I am now sleeping much better; another plus, not waking many times each night. As soon as I feel a hot flush starting I drink a small amount of water and it subsides. With so many women on HRT these days it would be good if this message could be included on your web-site. If you want any more information from me you can contact me on my email. Regards, M.

Heart attack; cardiovascular complications
Attestation: 25 March 1992

It was in the spring of 1991 when I first learned from a member of the Foundation For the Simple In Medicine the value of water as a form of medication. Six months before, I had suffered two heart attacks and had undergone angioplasty surgery. After the operation, I was prescribed heavy dosages of calcium and beta blockers, baby aspirin, nitroglycerine (for pain) and cholesterol-reducing medicine for recovery. The angiogram before the angioplasty had shown one of the arteries of my heart was 97 percent blocked by cholesterol deposits. I was told my heart had been damaged.

After six months of strict attention to my prescribed 'recuperation' program, I noticed that my condition was rapidly deteriorating, to the extent that I had difficulty sleeping because of pain in my left arm, back and chest, and also felt these same pains when I took my daily walks. I visualized myself going for bypass surgery at the scheduled time for re-evaluation of my condition. By this time, I also suffered from serious side-effects caused by the medications, such as: my

153

prostate created retention and blocking problems; I had also developed problems with my vision and memory recall.

I first began my rehabilitation through diet by a regular intake of six to eight 8-ounce glasses of water each day for three days. I was told to drink water a half-hour before eating my daily meals. I cut off my anti-cholesterol pills, aspirin and nitroglycerine pills. Judging by the effect of the water, it seemed I did not need them. I also started taking orange juice and started using salt in my diet again (I had been on a sodium-free diet). After the first three days, I was feeling more comfortable about all of that added water. After three weeks of gradually reducing the calcium and beta-blockers, I noticed some very favorable changes. Whenever I felt pain, I would drink water and get instant relief. My diet remained the same—fruits, vegetables, chicken, fish, orange juice, and carrot juice. To get more tryptophan, I was asked to add cottage cheese and lentil soup to my diet.

Dr. Batmanghelidj requested that I take two one-hour walks (25 min. mile) a day. After the second month, I noticed no more pain— even walking up steep hills. After the fifth month, I changed my walks to 1/2 hour and increased my pace to a 15-minute mile. No constrictions were noticed during my walks and my energy had increased two-fold. Much of my power to recall had been re-established, and my vision returned to normal.

In October 1991, I had a series of chemical and physical tests, including x-rays, sonogram, echocardiogram and electrocardiogram, to determine the state of my heart. The tests showed that my heart had restored to its normal state and I did not need any form of medication to cope with my daily routine. My doctor could not believe how simply all this change had taken place.

John O. Fox
Bates-Fox Natural Vision Training
Arlington, Virginia

Palpitations; false appendicitis pain; back pain, weight gain

Dear Phillip. It must be over 15 yrs since I read Dr Batman's *Your Bodies Many Cries For Water*. The information from this book has had a lasting impact on my life. At the time I suffered from 1) palpitations, 2) discomfort in the appendix area, 3) severe lower back pain and 4) weight gain. I decided to put Dr Batman's theory to the test. To my astonishment it WORKED!!! I went on to learn more about protecting my health and changed the direction of my life completely. I left behind my work in conventional medicine and went on to study natural healing, which I have been doing for the past 16 yrs. Madeline F-F, Athlone, Ireland

Dying of Thirst

I MUST be very naive. When my father died in a Midlands hospital last month, I suspected he had slowly become dehydrated over the three-and-a-half weeks he'd been in hospital. I had absolutely no idea that it is acknowledged widespread practice to deny drinking water to the elderly who are terminally ill (Letters). We had been taking a flask of tea to my father every afternoon, holding his cup for him. How he loved that drink. The nurses changed his water jug daily, but he couldn't physically pour from a jug. He could lift a cup and on one visit a cousin found him desperately trying to drink from an empty beaker. I was under the impression that access to clean drinking water is a basic right to life.

Ruth Dallaway, Wolverhampton, UK
Daily Mail, 18th February 2008

Weight loss

Dear Dr Batmanghelidj

My mother asked that I write to you and tell you about my recent weight loss success. I know that I could have a much more successful loss if I would follow your formula and curb my eating habits, along with starting a regular routine of exercise. However just getting myself to get off of six to eight cans of Mountain Dew a day is a miracle in itself.

Within the last nine months to a year, I have successfully been able to keep 35 excess pounds of baggage off. I am able to wear clothes that I thought would never touch my body again. I also have just about reached my goal size for my upcoming wedding. Even my fiancé had to admit that I am looking much better than when he first met me five years ago.

My success has been contributed to faithfully drinking half my body weight in ounces in water every day. Wherever I go, so does my water. To work, shopping, even my long seven-hour long car rides. (That does make for a lot of rest area stops, but they are worth it.) I do treat myself to an occasional mineral water or beer when I go out, but I have usually gotten my quota of water in for the day.

One interesting thing that I have noticed, however, is that once I have finished drinking my quota of water, I have absolutely no desire to drink anymore. Also I have found that I'm not thirsty anymore and it will usually take me awhile to drink some other type of beverage whether it be juice, milk, beer, mineral water, etc.

I am looking forward to October 1st which is my wedding day when I can walk down the aisle looking better than I have looked in 15 years, since I graduated from high school. It will also be nice to put my weight on my new driver's license without having to cringe for the first time in my life.

Thanks for the smaller me!!!! Donna G

Multiple Sclerosis

I've had MS for about 5 years. My symptoms included being confined to bed for a month, retaining fluid so badly that I couldn't walk and I weighed 175 lbs. Being short, it really showed up on me. I could hardly talk as well. I didn't know what was wrong with me at the time. My husband was concerned and didn't know what to do for me or with me. Another problem was that I had a chronic bladder condition. I have been to numerous doctors and hospitals in Canada, New York

City and Pennsylvania. I've had every test that has been written or given to find out what the problem was with my bowels and bladder. I was told that it was a condition that I had to learn to live with and would end up with a colostomy. I am an LPN and I've been a nurse for 44 years.

I've taken all kinds of medications prescribed for me, thinking they would help. I was diagnosed for sure with MS at Geisinger in Danville last March. They said that I have had MS for about 5 years. This last year it got to be severe.

I wasn't really following the Water Cure until it got very severe. My husband tried it and lost 40 lbs. in a month. Even his disposition and nervousness improved. All the medicine that I was taking, I stopped taking. I had seen such an improvement in my intellect, memory, coordination, breathing; upper respiratory problems were gone as well. My bowel and bladder were stagnated, but they now were starting to function the way they should.

I hadn't seen my doctor for a couple of months. When I walked in, he couldn't believe what he saw. "You look wonderful," is what he said to me. He asked what I was doing. I told him that I was on Dr. Batmanghelidj's Water Cure, the water and salt cure! He asked what that was all about. I told him that everyone needs to drink 2 quarts of water daily and add half a tsp. of salt as seasoning on their food. He said evidently it does work because he could see the results in me and said, Marilyn, you have never been in better health. He thinks it is the greatest thing he has ever heard.

His name is Dr. John Carey. He has an office here in Kingston and another in Dallas. He even tried it himself and has now lost a lot of weight thanks to the Water Cure. He said that this therapy is so simple and unique that it has to get out to the people. He has always been the type of doctor who believes in helping the individual patient doing whatever is good for the patient; it doesn't matter where it comes from. If it is good for them, he wants them to have it. Something tragic had to happen like Dr. Batmanghelidj being in the prison waiting to be shot to make this discovery. I had to get MS to be able to do what I am doing today, which is telling everyone about it. In the Bible, you see salt and water. If we would all eat and drink and do the things like Jesus did when he was on this earth, and we all know he drank water and we all know that he must have eaten salt. We are the salt of the earth, and if it was good enough for Him, it's got to be good enough for us.. This has SAVED MY LIFE! You have my permission to share this letter with any one you want. Sincerely, M.F.

Multiple Sclerosis

I have had MS since 1989. I had periods of partial paralysis and uncomfortable muscle tremors. Until I came down with MS, I had never drunk water, I lived on coffee, now I drink no coffee and water is my main drink. My girlfriend told me about the water cure in 1995 – I thought it was ridiculous. In April 1996 I went blind in one eye due to MS. I had no energy and just wanted to sleep. I was on the water cure for a week and a half when I noticed the change. By the end of three weeks my eyesight came back and all other symptoms disappeared and I was filled with an incredible energy I never had before. My doctor could not believe I got my sight back that fast. He never had that happen before. My doctor didn't even question me as to how I got better. My message for other MS sufferers: try the water cure and do not give up. Sincerely, B.V.L.

Headaches

For many years I suffered with headaches. I consulted doctors, neurologists, chiropractors and spent hundreds of dollars for head-scans and X-rays, all to no avail. At times only my faith in God kept me from wanting to die as I lay prone on my bed for days on end in pain.

No medication would ever stop the pain, it would just seem to run its course and then stop. I could never make any connection between my diet and the headaches, and the only pattern they seemed to follow was to always start a couple of hours after a meal. Then one day a friend told me he thought my headaches were caused because I never drank enough water. While I knew I didn't actually drink much water, I thought my herbal tea with fruit juices together with lots of fruits amply supplied my liquid requirements. Just three weeks later I was leafing through a health magazine when an advertisement for your book, 'Your Body's Many Cries for Water', just seemed to leap out at my eyes. I bought the magazine and sent for the book.

When it came, I eagerly read and re-read it to learn this new concept about water, and as I saw the errors in my drinking habits I quickly set about to righting them. Can anyone, without experiencing it for themselves, really understand what it is like to have usually pain-filled days changed to wonderful painless days when you can do the things you want to do, instead of being 'down with a headache'? Oh, such a blessing, for which I thank God continually!

It has taken months to properly hydrate my body, but now a headache is a now-and-again event instead of the norm. I thank a loving and caring God for leading me step by step to this wonderful truth. He no doubt tried to lead me a lot earlier but I was too blind to see. I thank you, doctor, for your great work and perseverance in bringing this truth to the people.

I lecture to adults at night classes on 'Better Food and Eating Habits' and I quickly gave one of my sessions entirely to the body's need for water. I have been able to help many people to better health and much less pain in their lives with this knowledge. A friend told me he was going into hospital in a few days time for stomach and ulcer treatment. I begged him to cancel this and try the water treatment you recommended.

He somewhat reluctantly did and was amazed and thankful to find his pains stop and in time, to know that the ulcer had healed, all without medication.

Please let me offer my grateful thanks again and pray that the Lord will bless and guide you and your staff as you work for the better health of humanity. Sincerely, Mavis B

Overweight, allergies, blood pressure and asthma:

This letter is a testimony to the merits of water as an essential part of the dairy dietary requirements for good health. I have been following your recommendations for nearly five years and have found myself taking for granted the positive effects of water intake.

When I first started on the program I was overweight, with high blood pressure and suffering from asthma and allergies, which I have had since a small child. I had been receiving treatment for these conditions. Today, I have my weight and blood pressure under control (weight loss of approximately 30 pounds and a 10 point drop in blood pressure). The program reduced the frequency of asthma and allergy related problems to the point of practical non-existence. Additionally, there were other benefits; I experienced fewer colds and flus, and generally with less severity.

I introduced this program to my wife, who had been on blood pressure medication for the past four years, and through increased water intake has recently bean able to eliminate her medication. Thanks again for your program. Michael P.

High blood pressure

Dear Dr. Batmanghelidj: I am in a position to verify how tap water effectively lowers hypertension. Starting in early April 1994, leaving years of diuretics and calcium-blockers behind, in accordance with your recommendation, for approximately 3 months I drank a minimum of eight 8-ounce glasses of tap water; occasionally more. The blood pressure, heretofore contained by drugs, gradually dropped from an average around 150-160 systolic/over 95-98 diastolic to an amazing, drug free, 130-135 systolic/over 75-80 diastolic fluctuating average.

My wife makes these measurements at home, each time taking two or three readings. The record shows several lows of 120s. over 75d. and a rare high of 140s. over 90d. However, the average range, as stated above, uniformly dominates.

In addition to vitamins and minerals, this drug-free approach, based essentially on water and a pinch of salt, has relaxed my systems and justifies the confidence that you hold the handles of a truly revolutionary and marvelous medical concept.

Since you are about to publish a book with applicable testimonies of the hydration system, my personal experience is gratefully offered as a way of saying thank you.

Lt. Col. W B (Ret)

Opinion

Thank you for your gifts! Your gift of knowledge is the best of all. Patients are now coming back for office visits after I have told them about water. They are getting better. I believed you, but it nice to get confirmation from patients. In general, I am very open-minded but I do not anticipate that any scientific evidence will arise to change my opinion.

Anyway, keep up the great work the Lord has given you. My work involves chronic Lyme disease, intestinal yeast, low metabolism bioelectric medicine and others. Your work is making mine easier. Thanks, **Charles L Crist, MD**

Do NOT drink fluoridated water!

Phillip Day: The term 'fluoride' is often used to describe fluorine-based chemical additives put into the public water supply or toothpastes and foods. 'Fluoride' tablets are also prescribed to youngsters apparently to assist in the protection and development of their teeth. In repeatedly hearing the one term, 'fluoride', the public has been cleverly persuaded to imagine there is just one substance that has been made available by caring government and industry to maintain and promote healthy teeth and gums. The reality is, the term 'fluoride' is used to encompass everything from sodium, calcium and potassium fluorides through to the highly dangerous liquid toxic waste product hexafluorosilicic acid and the toxic powder sodium silicofluoride, both of which are used to fluoridate water supplies.

Pure fluorine is gaseous and is described as 'a non-metallic halogen element that is isolated as a pale yellowish flammable irritating toxic diatomic gas' (Webster's Ninth New Collegiate Dictionary, 1991). Fluorine was used to great effect as a battlefield gas by the militaries during World War 1. Fluoride compounds today are used in pesticides, aluminium smelting, etching metals and glass, aerosol propellants and refrigerants. Sodium fluoride, the same compound that is added to toothpastes under the admiring eye of the world's dental associations, is a chief component of Sarin nerve gas. It's also the main ingredient in rat poison, as any pest control expert will tell you.

Is fluoride safe? You be the judge

> Fluoride accumulates in the body like lead, inflicting its damage over long periods of time. Fluoride is more toxic than lead, and slightly less toxic than arsenic. Lead is given a toxicity rating of 3, whereas fluoride's level is 4. Under US law, administered and enforced by the Environmental

Protection Agency, the maximum allowable lead in drinking water is 0.015mg/litre. With fluoride however it is 4.0mg/litre, *over 350 times the permitted lead level.* [17]

> Fluoride compounds initially cause dental fluorosis, a chalky mottling of the tooth enamel, leading to brittle and vulnerable teeth. Fluorosis is a permanent malformation of tooth enamel indicating an alteration in bone growth. Further symptoms of chronic fluoride poisoning may include constipation, excess gas and other gastrointestinal disturbances, chronic boils or rashes, peeling, shrivelled skin between your toes or brittle, easy-to-break nails. Symptoms of extreme fluoride poisoning may include chronic fatigue syndrome, skin problems, bleeding gums, excess saliva, hair loss, edema swelling in the lower extremities, mental problems, kidney disease and cancer.[18]

> *'The fluoride dose prescribed by doctors and the dose administered without prescription to everyone in community drinking water is EXPECTED to cause dental fluorosis in 10% of children. Actual Public Health Service figures show that 30% of children in fluoridated localities have dental fluorosis and 10% of children in non-fluoridated areas now have fluorosis.'*[19] Even citizens living in non-fluoridated areas are expected to ingest amounts in excess of 1.0mg fluoride compounds per day through toothpaste use and consumption of food products manufactured with fluoridated water. Citizens living in fluoridated communities <u>may expect to be exposed to 5.0mg a day or more.</u>

---

[17] *Clinical Toxicology of Commercial Products*, 5th Ed. 1984

[18] Dr Leo Spira's testimony before a US Senate investigative committee explained that the long-term effects of fluoride compound poisoning potentially implicated the chemical in a host of problems not readily identifiable as fluoride-causation, in view of the length of exposure.

[19] *Health Action Network* briefing document, op. cit. Also, *Review of Fluoride Benefits and Risks*, US Public Health Service, February 1991, p.53

- Medical research shows that hip fractures are 20-40% higher in fluoridated communities. [20]
- Fluorides are used in laboratory work to inhibit enzyme activity. Fluoride compounds have the same effect in the human body, accumulating in the skeleton structure over long periods of time. Fluoride poisoning is long-term and progressive.
- The chemicals injected into public water supplies to elevate fluoride levels are raw industrial waste. The real reason they are added is to dispose of toxic waste without millions of dollars/pounds in costs. The two most commonly used additives are hexafluorosilicic acid (H_2SIF_6) and sodium silicofluoride, toxic by-products of aluminium smelting and phosphate fertiliser production.
- Fluoridated water increases corrosion and leaching of lead from water mains and plumbing.
- About 1% of the fluoridated water used from public supplies is actually ingested by the public. The remainder is used for sewage, washing, industry and agriculture. This had led to the belief by industry that fluoridated industrial waste may be safely disposed of in this manner with little or no harm to the public. However, fluoride levels in the sewer effluent of fluoridated water systems are not monitored or controlled. Fish have been found to be poisoned by fluoride emissions at and below the 'acceptable' levels emitted by sewer effluent.[21]

Fluoridation - mass-medication without consent

Water fluoridation has been described as the widest mass-medication program in the history. That this procedure is occurring without the informed consent of the citizenry is the chief ethical issue

---

[20] *The John R Lee MD Medical Letter*, February 1999
[21] Health Action Network, op. cit.

driving opposition to fluoridation since World War 2. Researcher Janet Nagel summarises:

'That nearly all physicians, dentists and other members of the dominant health professions have come to hold such uncritical faith in fluoride as a tooth decay remedy raises serious questions about the content and quality of their training as scientists and practitioners. That so many professional leaders and government officials have been willing to falsify or obscure scientific data in their zeal to maintain the fluoridation pretense raises concerns that are even more far-reaching.' [22]

The charge of mass medication of the population can justifiably be made since fluoride is, by the admission of its proponents, pharmacologically active in supposedly preventing dental caries. Many of the trials quoted in my book *Health Wars* demonstrate inarguably that fluoride compounds are also pharmacologically active in doing human and animal systems harm. Even the Food & Drug Administration wishes the whole fluoride embarrassment would go away, having classified water fluoride compounds as 'unapproved new drugs' and obstinately left it at that. On the 16th March 1979, a surreptitious changing of the Federal Register occurred on page 16006. All paragraphs stating that fluoride compounds were 'essential or probably essential' were deleted by the FDA.

There are not many who will dispute the fact that fluoride compounds in amounts of 1.0 ppm (as advocated by fluoride proponents) do not produce changes in tooth enamel structure and bone formation (toothpaste fluoride concentrations are usually up around 1450 ppm!). The point being made by fluoride opponents is that the citizens themselves should have the right to decide whether or not to take fluoride supplementation. At the present time, there is no regulation as to how much fluoride any given individual is taking in,

---

[22] Ibid.

due to varied water consumption, age, occupation, diet and lifestyle. This has led to obvious concerns over health risks which have failed to disperse over the years, which only serve to underline more forcibly the unassailable conclusion that there are no known essential uses for fluoride compounds in medicine or dentistry.

As a last example of how even experts in the field of chemistry and medicine have remained divided on this issue over the years, the following Nobel Prize winners have either expressed reservations about fluoridation or outright opposed it:

Adolf Butenandt (Chemistry, 1939)
Arvid Carlsson (Chemistry, 2000)
Hans von Euler-Chelpin (Chemistry, 1929)
Walter Rudolf Hess (Medicine, 1949)
Corneille Jean-François Heymans (Medicine, 1938)
Sir Cyril Norman Hinshelwood (Chemistry, 1956)
Joshua Lederberg (Medicine, 1958)
William P. Murphy (Medicine, 1934)
Giulio Natta (Chemistry 1963)
Sir Robert Robinson (Chemistry, 1947)
Nikolai Semenov (Chemistry, 1956)
James B. Sumner (Chemistry, 1946)
Hugo Theorell (Medicine, 1955)
Artturi Virtanen (Chemistry, 1945)[23]

Dr John Lee summarises:

FACT 1
Fluoridation is cancer-causing, cancer-promoting, and is linked to increased cancer rates in humans.[24]

---

23 The Fluoridation Action Network, www.fluoridealert.org
24 *Carcinogenesis*, Vol. 9, 1988 pp.2279-2284; 'Sodium Fluoride; Individual Animal Tumor Pathology Table [rats], Battelle Memorial Institute, 23rd February 1989; *Lancet* 36 1990, p.737;

FACT 2

Hip fracture rates are substantially higher in people residing in fluoridated communities.[25]

FACT 3

Dental fluorosis, the first visible sign of fluoride poisoning, affects from 8% to 51% of the children drinking fluoridated water.[26]

FACT 4

All of the recent large-scale studies on fluoridation and tooth decay show that fluoridation *does not* reduce tooth decay.[27]

FACT 5

Fluoride drops and tablets are not approved by the US Food & Drug Administration as safe and effective. On the contrary, fluoride tablets and drops have been shown to be ineffective in reducing tooth decay and can cause skin eruptions, gastric distress, headache and weakness, which disappear when fluoride use is discontinued. Dental fluorosis on the other hand, is a permanent disfigurement.[28]

Conclusion

If you live in a fluoridated water zone and wish to drink tap water without fluoride, your supply will need to be fitted with a reverse osmosis filter system or better. RO systems are now quite reasonably

---

Review of Fluoride: Benefits and Risks, US Public Health Service, 1991, pp. F1-F7; *Fluoride*, Vol. 26, 1992, pp.83-96; *A Brief Report on the Association of Drinking Water Fluoridation and the Incidence of Osteosarcoma Among Young Males*, New Jersey Department of Health, November 1992; *Fluoride, the Aging Factor*, Health Action Press, 1993, pp.72-90

[25] *Journal of the American Medical Association (JAMA)*, Vol. 264, 1990, pp.500-502; *JAMA*, Vol. 266, 1991, pp.513-514; *JAMA*, Vol. 268, 1992, pp.746-748; *JAMA*, Vol. 273, 1995, pp. 775-776

[26] *Science*, Vol. 217, 1982, pp.26-30; *Journal of the American Dental Association*, Vol. 108, 1984, pp.56-59; *Journal of Public Health Dentistry*, Vol. 46, 1986, pp.184-187; *Health Effects of Ingested Fluoride*, National Research Council, 1993, p.37

[27] *Community Health Studies*, Vol. 11, 1987, pp.85-90; *Journal of the Canadian Dental Association*, Vol. 53, 1987, pp.763-765; *Fluoride*, Vol. 23, 1990, pp.55-67

[28] Letter from Frank R Fazzari, Chief, Prescription Drug Compliance, US Food & Drug Administration to New Jersey Assemblyman John Kelly, 8th June 1993; *Preventing Tooth Decay: Results from a Four-Year National Study*, Robert Wood-Johnson Foundation, Special Report #2/1983, 18 pages; *Community Dentistry and Oral Epidemiology*, Vol. 19, 1991, pp.88-92; *1992 Physicians Desk Reference*, p.2273

priced and can be installed with average DIY experience.[29] They will clean the water down to 15-30 ppm, taking out fluoride, chlorine, estrogens, trihalomethanes, nitrates and medications, leaving the water with a small mineral content to ensure stability. Avoid drinking distilled water, which has been linked to heart damage and strokes.[30] Bottled water is OK if a little expensive. Avoid drinking water out of warm, flexible plastic bottles as chemicals can be emitted which mimic estrogen.

* * * * *

Warning label on US toothpastes: *Warning! In case of accidental ingestion, seek professional help or contact a poisons control center immediately.*

Warning label on UK toothpastes: *Use a pea-sized amount.*

---

[29] www.credence.org sells the Pura-Flow reverse osmosis drinking water system. If you live outside the EU, RO systems are available from DIY stores or specialist suppliers. More expensive granulated filters are also available. Avoid drinking high alkalised water, which can cause problems over the long-term.

[30] www.mercola.com

Common alkali ash foods
(Help to control acid in your internal environment)

Almonds
Apples
Apricots
Avocados
Bananas
Beans, dried
Beet greens
Beet
Blackberries
Broccoli
Brussels sprouts
Cabbage
Carrots
Cauliflower
Celery
Chard leaves
Cherries, sour
Cucumbers
Dates, dried
Figs, dried
Grapefruit
Grapes
Green beans
Green peas
Lemons
Lettuce

Milk, goat*
Millet
Molasses
Mushrooms
Muskmelons
Onions
Oranges (small portions)
Parsnips
Peaches
Pears
Pineapple (small portions)
Potatoes, sweet
Potatoes, white
Radishes
Raisins
Raspberries
Rutabagas
Sauerkraut
Soy beans, green
Spinach, raw
Strawberries
Tangerines
Tomatoes
Watercress
Watermelon

* Recommended for infants only when mother's milk is not available.

Note: Some of the above foods may seem acidic but leave an alkali ash in the system. Convert your diet to 80% alkali ash/20% acid ash foods. Ensure that your diet is predominantly high-water content foods that are fresh and organic. Supplementation with trace minerals, fish oils and vitamins is also recommended.

Common acid ash foods

Bacon
Barley grain
Beef
Blueberries
Bran, wheat
Bran, oat
Bread, white
Bread, whole wheat
Butter
Carob
Cheese
Chicken
Cod
Corn
Corned beef
Crackers, soda
Cranberries
Currants
Eggs
Flour, white
Flour, whole wheat
Haddock
Lamb
Lentils, dried
Lobster
Milk, cow's ^

Macaroni
Oatmeal
Oysters
Peanut butter
Peanuts
Peas, dried
Pike
Plums ^
Pork
Prunes ^
Rice, brown
Rice, white
Salmon
Sardines
Sausage
Scallops
Shrimp
Spaghetti
Squash, winter
Sunflower seeds
Turkey
Veal
Walnuts
Wheat germ
Yoghurt

^ These foods leave an alkaline ash but have an acidifying effect on the body.

NEUTRAL ASH FOODS THAT HAVE AN ACIDIFYING EFFECT

Corn oil   Corn syrup   Olive oil   Refined sugar

Contacts

If you wish to purchase more copies of this book or any of Credence's other book and disk products, please use the contact details below. Credence has local sales offices in several countries. Our website at www.credence.org can give you further details:

> UK Orders: (01622) 832386
> UK Fax: (01622) 833314
> www.credence.org
> e-mail: sales@credence.org

Credence Publications
PO Box 3
TONBRIDGE
Kent TN12 9ZY
England
sales@credence.org

THE CAMPAIGN FOR TRUTH IN MEDICINE

Once a month, the Campaign for Truth in Medicine sends out the EClub Internet bulletin to thousands of subscribers worldwide. This informative e-mail newsletter is available FREE to customers who have purchased this book or requested EClub. This online bulletin contains the latest news and research on cancer, heart disease, mental health and other health topics. *Do not be without this great resource!* To subscribe for free, log on to www.campaignfortruth.com and click the 'Join CTM' tab to complete your application.

Index

Kent, England, 178
Kii, Japan, 61
Kinins, 24
Koran, 18

L

Le Fanu, Dr James, 5
Lepitin, 92
Libido, 38, 45, 61, 140, 144
Lipase, 81, 82
Lipton, Dr Bruce, 17
Lithium, 43
Liver, 27, 34, 70, 75, 80, 81, 83, 101, 113,
130, 133, 139, 142, 144
Lourdes, 18
Lymph, 124

M

McLeod, Prof Malcolm, 103
Melatonin, 43, 45, 98, 102, 138, 143
Mercola, Dr Joseph, 38
Methionine, 96, 97, 100
Migraine, 11, 109, 110
Morning sickness, 11, 21, 144
Motilin, 64, 88, 99
Multiple sclerosis (MS), 31, 97, 137, 144
Music, 29, 124, 125

N

Nagel, Janet, 165
National Library of Medicine,
Bethesda, 48
Neck pain, 108
New England Journal of Medicine, 77
New Jersey, USA, 167
Neways, 122
Nobel Prize, 166

Noradrenaline, 82, 139

O

Obesity, 35, 80
Overweight, 11, 91, 160

P

Pancreas, 13, 64, 127, 128, 129, 130, 136
Parkinson's disease, 139
Peppermint, 123
Peristalsis, 64, 65
Phospholipids, 83
Potassium, 32, 40, 41, 42, 46, 51, 97, 98,
99, 123, 126, 127, 128, 132, 162
Prolactin, 117
Prostaglandins, 24
Psychiatry, 96
Psychology, 96
Pyloric valve, 63, 64, 65

R

Rat poison, 162
Renin-angiotensin, 24
Rockefeller, John, 4

S

Saliva, 13, 45, 92, 163
Sarin, 162
Schiff, Moritz, 12
Selenium, 122, 123
Serotonin, 43, 45, 88, 96, 98, 99, 100,
101, 102, 126, 138, 143
Sheldrake, Dr Rupert, 17
Simoncini, Dr Tullio, 122
Sodium fluoride, 162
Sodium silicofluoride, 162, 164

Sunlight, 124

Reflections

Then the men of the city said to Elisha, "Please notice the situation of this city is pleasant, as my lord sees; but the water is bad, and the ground barren." And he said, "Bring me a new bowl and put salt in it." So they brought it to him. Then he went out to the source of the water and cast in the salt there and said, "Thus says the Lord, I have healed this water; from it there shall be no more death or barrenness." So the water remains healed to this day, according to the word of Elisha which he spoke. **2 Kings 2:19-22**

Should you not know that the Lord God of Israel gave the dominion of Israel to David forever, to him and his sons, by a covenant of salt? **2 Chronicles 13:5**

Jesus said, "You are the salt of the earth; but if the salt loses its flavour, how shall it be seasoned? It is then good for nothing but to be thrown out and trampled underfoot by men." **Matthew 5:13**

Jesus said, "Salt is good, but if the salt loses its flavour, how will you season it? Have salt in yourselves, and have peace with one another." **Mark 9:50**

About the Authors

Dr Fereydoon Batmanghelidj – known as 'Dr Batman' or simply 'Dr B' to his ever-widening international audience – has successfully treated thousands of patients simply by using water. Born in Iran in 1931, he was educated in Scotland at Fettes School. Later he studied medicine under Sir Alexander Fleming, the discoverer of penicillin, at London University. He practised medicine in Tehran until 1979, when he was imprisoned and sentenced 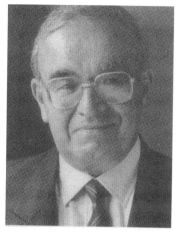 to death along with many other innocent Iranians during the violent revolution that overthrew the Shah. While in prison he discovered the healing powers of plain water by prescribing a single glass for a prisoner dying of acute stomach pain. Pardoned because of his discovery, he was released in 1982 and escaped to the United States, where he set up the Foundation for the Simple in Medicine to explore and communicate his discovery that dehydration is the true cause of many illnesses. He is the bestselling author of *Your Body's Many Cries for Water* and other related books including *Water Cures, Drugs Kill; Eradicate Asthma Now - with Water,* and *How to Deal With Back Pain and Rheumatoid Joint Pain.*

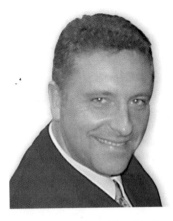

Phillip Day was born in England in 1960 and educated at Selwyn and Charterhouse. Throughout his twenties, he enjoyed a successful entrepreneurial career in business and became interested in wars going on in the realms of health and politics after overcoming his own health problems.

Today, Phillip Day heads up Credence Publications and is founder of the global citizen's advocacy group, The Campaign for Truth in Medicine. For many years he has been a staunch supporter of Dr Batmanghelidj's work and speaks to thousands around the world each year on disease, medical quackery and the importance of the citizen taking control over their own life. He has written thirteen books on health, including the best-selling *Cancer: Why We're Still Dying to Know the Truth, Health Wars, Simple Changes* and the award-winning *The Mind Game*. He has appeared as a citizen's champion on TV, radio and in documentaries around the world where these subjects are aired. Phillip's intention is to work with the establishments and organisations concerned to resolve issues that are harming the public, and to provide the necessary information for citizens to make their own informed choices. He is married to Samantha and lives in Kent, England.